Praise for *Outsmarting the Midlife Fat Cell*

"Debra has done it again—but this time for us baby boomers who are now finding out firsthand about what our mothers referred to as 'the change,' including changes in our fat cells. Debra shows that these changes can be handled with humor, a positive attitude—and some chocolate-covered strawberries!"
—Carol Johnson, author of *Self-esteem Comes in All Sizes: How to Be Happy and Healthy at Your Natural Weight*

"Required reading for all women anticipating, experiencing, or recalling their menopause!"
—Laurel Mellin, author of *The Solution* and associate professor of medicine, University of California, San Francisco

"Debra Waterhouse has done it again—she has written an important book that is long overdue. Waterhouse shatters the weight enigma with menopause and makes a compelling argument on how dieting only worsens the transition. More importantly, she takes a 'meno-positive' approach on how to manage weight without dieting, especially during the critical preceding years that begin at about age 35. A must read."
—Evelyn Tribole, M.S., R.D., co-author of *Intuitive Eating*

"Debra Waterhouse's exploration of the physical changes of menopause finally offers some clarity—and hope—for women who grew up in the diet culture. Her program proposes moderation, good sense, and self-acceptance in a time when all three are sorely lacking."
—Michelle Stacey, author of *Consumed: Why Americans Love, Hate, and Fear Food*

"This down-to-earth inspirational book gives the midlife woman sound advice for developing a healthy body and body image. Perhaps more important is the underlying optimistic and empowering philosophy that midlife is a natural and positive phase of life."
—Carol Landau, Ph.D.,
author of *The Complete Book of Menopause*

"Waterhouse brilliantly customizes *Outsmarting the Midlife Fat Cell* for menopausal women. Information is power, and Waterhouse arms women with a wealth of weight information at one of the most challenging times of their lives."
—Elaine Magee, M.P.H., R.D.,
author of *Eat Well for a Healthy Menopause*

"At a time when the shelves are filled with a never-ending stream of fad diet books based on myth and misconception, it is refreshing to read a book based on practical, trustworthy, and useful information—advice that has worked for thousands of women and that encourages us to listen to our bodies, trust our eating instincts, and tap into our bodies' food wisdom."
—Elizabeth Somer, M.A., R.D.

"The book is wonderful! It appeals to midlife women's concerns about weight gain, but it then, in a very well-researched style, elucidates the reasons women should avoid dieting and focus on self-acceptance and health. As a psychotherapist and an eating disorders prevention consultant to schools, professional organizations, and universities, I am seeing an increase in the incidence of disordered eating in midlife women. I am very pleased to see a book that so thoroughly and professionally addresses women's concerns and offers a program that will lead to self-esteem, confidence, and health into old age!"
—Elizabeth Scott, L.C.S.W.,
eating disorders prevention consultant

Outsmarting the Midlife Fat Cell

Also by Debra Waterhouse, M.P.H., R.D.

Outsmarting the Female Fat Cell
Why Women Need Chocolate
Like Mother, Like Daughter

Outsmarting the
Midlife Fat Cell

Winning Weight Control Strategies for Women Over

5 to Stay Fit Through Menopause

DEBRA WATERHOUSE, M.P.H., R.D.

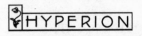

New York

The advice in this book is not intended for persons with chronic illnesses or other conditions that may be worsened by an unsupervised eating and/or exercise program. The recommendations are not intended to replace or conflict with advice given to you by your physician or other health professional, and we recommend that you do consult with your physician. The author and publisher cannot be held responsible for any results arising from use or application of the information in this book.

Except for those who have given permission to appear in this book, all names in this book have been changed. In some cases, composite accounts have been created based on the author's professional experience.

Page 233, "An Apology to My Body" reprinted with permission from the author, Marlena Gutierrez.

Copyright © 1998, Debra Waterhouse, M.P.H., R.D.
All rights reserved. No part of this book may be used or reproduced in any manner whatsoever without the written permission of the Publisher. Printed in the United States of America. For information address: Hyperion, 114 Fifth Avenue, New York, New York 10011.
Library of Congress Cataloging-In-Publication Data
Waterhouse, Debra.
    Outsmarting the midlife fat cell : winning weight control strategies for women over 35 to stay fit through menopause / Debra Waterhouse. — 1st ed.
      p.   cm.
    Includes bibliographical references and index.
    ISBN 0–7868–6284–X
    1. Weight loss.   2. Middle aged women—Health and hygiene.
3. Middle aged women—Nutrition 4. Menopause. I. Title.
RM222.2.W7285   1998
613.2'5—dc21   97–46937
                                            CIP

FIRST EDITION
10 9 8 7 6 5 4 3
Designed by Robert Bull Design

To my sister and best friend
Lori Waterhouse Erwin
who radiates beauty inside and out

Acknowledgments

My life is blessed with an extraordinary support system filled with colleagues, friends, clients, and family, almost all of whom have been by my side for the writing of four books. My greatest support person is my sister, Lori Waterhouse Erwin, who has been my writing anchor and reader-on-demand, selflessly enduring hundreds of calls, faxes, E-mails, and overnight deliveries. I not only owe a world of thanks to her, but also her three adorable sons, Timothy, Max, and Luke, whose precious voices never failed to dissolve writer's block and calm deadline stress.

Keeping with the theme of calming voices, my gifted editor, Judith Riven, had an endless supply of encouragement and insight. Her expertise and wisdom are reflected in every page of this book.

I applaud my agent, Sandra Dijkstra, along with her associates Rita Holm and Steve Malk, for their unfailing commitment to me and belief in my work. And I salute all at Hyperion, especially Bob Miller, Lisa Kitei, Tracey George, and Laurie Abkemeier for their unique dedication to their authors.

Special acknowledgment also goes to my circle of family, friends, and colleagues who eagerly donated valuable time to read my manuscript: Laura Euphrat; Laura Manca; Stephanie Goulding, R.N.; Dr. Dee Tivenan, M.F.C.C.; Dr. Kevin Tivenan; Dr. Elizabeth Markley Holm, R.D.; Dr. Catherine Christie, R.D.; Jeannette Highton Stansbury; Chrisi Kotis Brown, P.T.; Lisa VanDyke Euphrat; Mary Pat Cedarleaf; Joyce Gardiner Filatreau; Michelle Labadie Hawkins; Cheryl Winfield Bull; Mary Jane Arnold; and Amanda Kearney.

The book-writing process is immensely rewarding, but at times can also be isolating and frustrating. My husband, Paul Manca, provided his wonderful sense of humor to keep me smiling during the more difficult times, and my mother, Alina Waterhouse, instinctively knew when I needed a phone call to break up my day.

You all contributed greatly to this book as well as to my life. Thank you!

Contents

APPENDIXES

ATTENTION ALL 35- TO 55- YEAR-OLD WOMEN:

Why You Should Read This Book

*M*enopausal *weight gain*—it's real, it's necessary, and it's the most stubborn weight gain you'll ever experience. It's more stubborn than the weight you gained during pregnancy, and it's as essential as the weight you gained during puberty. It also starts when you're younger than you'd ever imagine and lasts longer than you'd like.

You may be in your mid 30s when the first few pounds mysteriously appear regardless of how little you've eaten or how much you've exercised, in your mid 40s when you come to the disheartening realization that your waist is two inches wider and your body is a full size larger, or in your mid 50s as you wonder if and when it's ever going to stop. Whether your midlife weight gain is just beginning or finally tapering off, you are among the *50 million* frustrated women who are crying out for help with their expanding waistlines and changing bodies.

This book is the answer to your universal cry for help—providing the knowledge, understanding, and solutions necessary to manage this mysterious weight gain and outsmart your midlife fat cells.

If you are in your mid 30s to early 40s, your initial reaction may be one of shock and resistance, "But I still have my periods and I don't have hot flashes! I can't possibly be in midlife! I'm too young to be menopausal!" The average woman lives to be about 80 years old, so the midway point is age forty—marking midlife. And, although you are probably too young to be *menopausal,* you're not too young to be just entering the transition to menopause, or as it's called now, *perimenopause.* Menopause is the clinical term used to mark the end of your menstrual cycles, but perimenopause refers to the years surrounding that event. Not just a couple of years, or a few years, but up to 20 years beforehand. Research is finding that this transition starts in the mid to late 30s for most women and ends in their mid 50s. That's one quarter of our lives!

But most women still think that menopause involves only a two- to four-year transition. While it's true that the most intense part of our transition lasts a few years, the initial changes begin more than a decade earlier when ever-so-slight hormonal changes affect your periods, moods, and weight. Your premenstrual symptoms begin to transform from moderate tension to "PMS from hell," your mood swings start to become mood sweeps, and your body shape progressively changes from an hourglass to a beer glass. You may have struggled with your weight before, but now the pounds accumulate without any appreciable change in your eating or exercise habits. If you are experiencing a change in your body shape, then you *are* in perimenopause and need to work with that reality.

The truth is: Your body changes before you technically enter "the change," and your *30 billion female fat cells* enter the menopausal transition before you do.

Each and every one of us has 30 billion fat cells, and a few years ago, research finally validated what we had long suspected: fat cells have gender. A woman's fat cells are physiologically different from a man's. They are larger, more active, and more resistant to dieting. And based on that long-awaited research, I wrote my first book, *Outsmarting the Female Fat Cell*, to provide a nondieting solution to weight loss that works with a woman's fat-storing physiology. At the end of *Outsmarting the Female Fat Cell*, I cautioned women that when they reach perimenopause, they will most likely have to outsmart their fat cells again.

Well, now you've reached that transition, and once again research is starting to surface to provide a physiological explanation for why female fat cells grow even larger and more stubborn during midlife. Here's a brief explanation: As soon as your fat cells detect a slightly lower estrogen level, they come to your aid to produce estrogen for you. (Fat cells producing estrogen? This may surprise you, but it's one of their highly evolved functions.) They know that eventually your ovaries will stop producing estrogen, so they start preparing to take over the ovaries' job. They increase their size, number, and ability to store fat. Interestingly enough, the fat cells in your waist grow the largest because they are better equipped to produce estrogen than the fat cells in your buttocks, hips, and thighs. The larger and more active your abdominal fat cells become, the more estrogen will be produced, and the more benefits you will receive: fewer hot flashes, milder mood swings, less intense PMS, improved sleep, a reduced risk of osteoporosis, and an overall easier transition. This is why larger women have always reported less menopausal stress while leaner women have the most difficulty with the transition.

Ironically, the very weight gain we abhor is actually beneficial for us. While we are waging war against our fat cells, they are looking out for our menopausal well-being.

You deserve to know, understand, and accept what's happening to your body and why it *has* to happen. You also are entitled to learn how to work successfully with your fat-storing physiology to achieve a healthy weight and a fit body.

Why hasn't anyone told you this before? Because most people, including health professionals, don't know. Hundreds of menopause books line the shelves of the women's health sections in bookstores, yet I couldn't find one that explained midlife weight gain physiologically or offered the guidance to manage it effectively. Instead, menopausal weight gain has been viewed as a part of the aging process and a result of eating too much and/or exercising too little. So the standard recommendation has been to eat less, exercise more, and diet harder to lose weight.

The harder you try to lose weight by dieting, the more powerful your menopausal fat cells will become, and the more weight you will gain. Diets don't work for most women regardless of age, but for menopausal women, diets have close to a 100 percent failure rate. Even on an 800-calorie diet, your fat cells will refuse to shrink and will fight back by growing even larger. Fat cells have an important mission of manufacturing estrogen and balancing your body during the transition—and they will do *everything* possible to make sure that they don't let you down.

If fat cells are invaluable for helping to ease the transition, then why are women reporting more menopausal discomfort, hot flashes, and forgetfulness than ever before? The headlines have informed us that obesity is on the rise and that women weigh more than ever, so what's going on? Are fat cells sleeping on the job? Have they lost their ability to produce estrogen? Our fat cells are not responsible; we are. We are preventing them from doing their job by interfering with their mission. Since puberty, we've dieted. We've skipped meals; skimped on carbos, fat, and sugar; and subjected our bodies to fasting, fad diets, liquid diets, and diet pills. Our fat cells have been so busy fighting our drastic weight loss attempts that they don't have the energy or resources left to manufacture estrogen and bring our bodies back into balance. Our fat cells are stressed out, and as a result, we're experiencing what I call "megamenopause."

Our transition is magnified compared to generations past. We are gaining 50 percent more weight than our mothers did, and our transition is 500 percent longer. We have more hot flashes, more memory loss, more insomnia, more everything. And most of the blame goes to dieting. Our mothers may have experimented with a few diets, but we declared dieting our life-long career.

Most women who are in midlife today started dieting in their teens and have been on at least fifteen diets, losing and re-gaining the same ten, twenty, or fifty pounds. Each time we di-eted, our estrogen levels dropped and our cortisol levels (one of the stress hormones) rose. After years of yo-yo dieting and yo-yoing hormones, our systems eventually wore out. The result: a longer transition, a more severe experience, and more weight gain.

Needless to say, this is not a book that outlines a "diet" to lose weight, nor does it guarantee getting your 20-year-old body back. This is a book that guarantees a full understanding of your female body during this important transition in your life—and guarantees that you will not gain more weight than is necessary and healthy for you.

This "minimizing weight gain" approach would not make it on the infomercial circuit or on the cover of a tabloid, but that's not my goal. Instead, my goal is to help you find your new natural healthy weight, prevent too much weight gain, lose weight if you've already gained too much, and accept this im-portant and fascinating stage of female passage. If you don't ac-cept it but choose to fight it through dieting, you'll only gain more weight, negatively influence your health, and have a more difficult transition.

As a registered dietitian in private practice, I have been counseling women for over sixteen years, and no other group is more confused and frustrated with their weights as those in peri-menopause. I've witnessed the pain they are in, but I have also witnessed the relief they feel when they come to a full and un-complicated understanding of why they are gaining weight and discover what they can do to manage it realistically.

In the following chapters, I will share with you what has been instrumental in helping over two thousand of my clients. Through years of analysis and research (and a little bit of trial and error), I have uncovered the attitudes and habits necessary to outsmart midlife fat cells. I call it "The Meno-Positive Approach to a Trimmer Transition." As your body is changing during the transition, your attitudes, eating habits, exercise habits, and lifestyle have to change along with it. By working with your new menopausal physiology, this plan highlights the positive actions you can take to keep midlife weight gain to a minimum (or lose weight if you've already gained too much) while at the same time allowing your fat cells to produce estrogen and bring your body back into balance. To accomplish this goal, The Meno-Positive Approach targets five essential steps:

1. **Acquiring meno-positive attitudes.** Your feelings about the transition, your body, and your weight affect your experience. Those women who have the most positive attitudes going into the transition have the least amount of weight gain and other potential problems by the time they come out of the transition. I'll help you initiate a positive attitude for your change in life, embrace your body changes, and manage your midlife weight crisis without dieting.

2. **Mastering meno-positive fitness.** Exercise is second only to attitudes in how you transition through menopause. Those women who exercise regularly gain only one half the weight of those who are sedentary, but your exercise program *must* be tailored to work specifically for menopause. I'll show you how to lose fat, gain muscle, increase your metabolism, strengthen your bones, and make your midlife fat cells fit.

3. **Embracing meno-positive eating habits.** How you structure your eating, when you eat, how often you eat, and how much you eat can either cause more fat storage or less. Because menopausal

women are highly efficient fat storers, we must modify our eating behavior to match our new midlife metabolism.

4. **Maximizing meno-positive food choices.** What you eat can also affect your transition and how much weight you gain. The focus is not on reducing calories and fat, it's on increasing phyto-estrogens (plant sources of estrogen), responding to your food cravings, and trusting your body's food messages. You'll learn how to eat well for "a change"—for managing hot flashes, fatigue, sleep, and mood swings.

5. **Living a meno-positive lifestyle.** In addition to eating and exercising, other lifestyle choices can positively affect your midlife years and your weight. Taking care of your body, managing stress, setting aside time for relaxation or meditation, and adding laughter and happiness to your life can all have a powerful effect on how you feel and function each day.

By focusing on fitness instead of thinness, you will minimize weight gain while maximizing well-being. With The Meno-Positive Approach, you will replace negative attitudes and habits with positive ones and learn how to:

- boost your metabolism, recharge your battery, and feel your best
- tame your fat cells, call a truce with food, and triumph with fitness
- throw away your scale, but not your common sense
- give up dieting, but not your desire to be healthy, fit, and strong
- let go of control, but not your commitment to taking care of yourself

After years of trying to control our female bodies—our emotions, weight, body shape, eating habits, and food intake—many of us now strive to control our bodies during menopause and remain unchanged during a time of immense change. We want to prevent menopause like we want to prevent osteoporosis, heart disease, or breast cancer. Well, it can't be prevented; it can only be experienced.

When women are asked the rhetorical question, "If you had a choice, would you rather not go through menopause?" most answer "no." We'd have to worry about contraception, cramps, tampons, pads, PMS, water retention, childbearing, and child rearing for the rest of our lives. We instinctively know that menopause keeps us healthy and alive. So let your body transition to menopause and allow it to find its new natural weight. It's only trying to help you find a healthy balance for the second half of your life. Give your body the freedom to find that balance and it will give you back so much more.

In this thin-worshipping, youth-oriented society, it may initially be difficult to take this positive, accepting approach. But if you don't, you will only gain more weight and become more weight preoccupied.

Haven't you spent enough of your life going on and off diets and feeling uncomfortable with your body? I always thought growth and maturity were supposed to free us from these superficial obsessions, but that's not what's happening. As we enter the transition to menopause, we are becoming more weight preoccupied and food obsessed. Think about it: women are entering perimenopause at an astronomical rate. Every day another 4,000 women embark on the journey, and 50 million women are gaining an average of 12 pounds—that's 600 million pounds of cumulative weight gain and 600 million pounds of weight preoccupation holding us down. We're already seeing the negative signs of this mass body dissatisfaction. Menopausal women represent one of the fastest growing segments of eating disorders and one of the fastest growing consumers of prescription diet pills. Here's another telltale sign: Researchers were funded last year to study women who have a positive body image during menopause and how that affects their transition, but they couldn't find enough women even to start the study!

Negative attitudes toward our bodies during menopause started in the 1950s when some doctors actually treated midlife women with tranquilizers. Then in the 1960s, from the best-selling book *Feminine Forever*, we learned from a gynecologist that menopause was an ominous marker of lost youth and a disease of estrogen deficiency. Unfortunately, this way of thinking continues today. A recent survey found that 53 percent of us consider menopause a medical condition that requires treatment. If you are one of those 53 percent, I hope that this introduction has triggered you to question your attitude and that the rest of this book will turn you completely around. ***Menopause is not a disease to be treated; it's a natural transition to be experienced.***

Is puberty a disease? No. Is pregnancy a disease? No. Puberty and pregnancy are healthy stages of female passage—and so is menopause. Like puberty, menopause is a shift in hormones, but in reverse. With the exception of hot flashes, menopause is the mirror image of puberty, and like puberty, the transition will end—weight will stabilize, moods will even out, and thinking will clear. You got through puberty without the benefit of years of wisdom and maturity. You'll get through menopause more smoothly if you let your wisdom and maturity guide you.

We *can* take a more positive approach to menopause and the weight gain associated with it, and we *can* change the way society views menopause. We've had a positive impact on society before, and we can do it again. As we moved through the previous stages of female passage, we changed them. We changed society's view of menstruation and PMS. We altered the birth control and childbirth industry. Now, we have an even stronger collective voice to change society's outlook on menopause.

But how will we change it? Will we keep dieting, fighting our bodies, and trying to defy biology? Or will we keep demanding research, going to conferences, surfing the Internet, and reading books to gather knowledge about what our bodies need to do during this important time in our lives?

My guess (and I'd bet a million dollars that I'm right) is that we will be proactive information gathers rather than self-destructive fighters. It's a part of who we are. When I shared with my husband that I thought I was entering the midlife transition with my mega-PMS and change in body shape, he jokingly said to me, "My advice, Deb, is to take it like a man. Just grin and bear it, and forget about it." Knowing he was trying to get a rise out of me, I immediately retorted, "No, I'll take it like a woman. I'll question it, research it, talk to my doctor about it, talk to my mother about it, talk to my friends about it, then talk about it some more to understand and manage it the best I can."

This book will give you all the research, education, facts, understanding, guidance, and solutions you'll need—so that we can all manage midlife weight gain and take menopause like "a woman."

chapter one

SO THAT'S WHY I'M GAINING WEIGHT!

Have you recently looked in the mirror and wondered where that extra body fat was coming from? Or tried on a pair of pants that you haven't worn for a couple of months only to discover you can't button the waist even with the previously successful lie-on-the-bed maneuver? Or gotten on the scale saying, "This can't be right; I couldn't possibly have gained four pounds in a week"?

When you honestly look at your eating and exercise habits, you are confident that you're not eating more or exercising less. Sure, you slipped a few times and ate real, luscious ice cream yesterday or a second helping of lasagna last week, but that can't possibly be the reason. Neither can a decrease in your activity level because you either don't exercise at all or you have a personal trainer who will vouch for your consistency.

Unable to figure out what's happening to your body, you make an appointment with your doctor for a complete medical exam. Your tests show that you are in perfect health. Still perplexed, you call your mother asking if adult onset obesity runs in your family. She tells you no and that you're probably imagining things. Then, you start talking to your friends, wondering if they, too, are experiencing this mysterious weight gain. They are, but they don't know why either.

This first chapter will piece together the mysterious puzzle of midlife weight gain by providing a full and uncomplicated explanation of how and why you are gaining weight. I can assure you that it's not the ice cream, the second helping of lasagna, or a missed exercise class, and chances are, it's not a physical ailment or a latent obesity gene either. It's **menopause**, and you are definitely not alone. Fifty million other women share your confusion and frustration.

If you are a fertile, hot flash–free 35- or 40-year-old woman, you may have flinched at the boldface **"M"** word. Let me clarify. You are still menstruating, so you are not menopausal in the classic sense and probably won't experience the hot flashes, memory loss, and other telltale signs for another decade or more. But you are entering the initial phase of menopause. You are entering perimenopause, the important ten- to twenty-year transition leading up to menopause, where your waist expands and your fat cells enlarge to prepare your body for the rest of the transition and the rest of your life.

Whether you are 35 and just about to enter the transition or 55 and just ending it, the good news is that you can take a deep breath and stop blaming yourself or your eating habits for this midlife weight gain. Researchers around the world have proven that an increase in calories, carbohydrates, fat, or alcohol does not explain menopausal body changes. But changes in hormonal levels, metabolism, and fat cell physiology do.

You are gaining weight because your fat cells are responding to lower hormonal levels, a drop in metabolism, and an overriding need to maintain your physical and emotional health during the menopausal transition and beyond. You may not want to gain weight (what woman does?), but your body wants to. You may think the best way to fight expanding fat cells is through dieting, but as you'll discover, your fat cells fight back now more than ever and will make you gain even more weight. The *only* way to manage menopausal weight permanently is to forgo dieting and begin a new, natural way of eating and exercising that works with your midlife fat cells instead of against them.

I'm not going to lead you to believe that you can turn back the clock and get back your 20-year-old body. You can't. The changes in your midlife body are biologically necessary and too important for your well-being to prevent them completely. But you *can* make your fat cells smaller and achieve a fit, healthy body by following a weight-control program designed specifically for menopause. However, before you can master this program, you need to know exactly what's happening to your body and fat cells during the transition. Before I can outline how to outsmart your midlife fat cells, I need to explain why they are so smart and stubborn to begin with. Because this knowledge will be both motivating and empowering, I'm going to first make you an expert in female fat cell physiology.

THE LIFE CYCLE OF A FEMALE FAT CELL

Each of your 30 billion female fat cells (that's right, 30 billion!) came into this world programmed with specific instructions. As soon as they figured out that they were female with two X chromosomes, they knew that they would have an exciting life ahead of them filled with activity and opportunity. They would have the power to store fat every single day, but especially during the three stages of female passage: puberty, pregnancy, and the transition to menopause.

I realize that puberty seems like a lifetime ago, and any pregnancies may be in the past (or maybe not, since more women are having children during perimenopause), but it's important to understand the specialized function of female fat cells throughout your life. The survival of the human race is dependent on our efficient, smart, stubborn fat cells that were activated at puberty, given more power with pregnancy, and then turbocharged during perimenopause.

Do you remember what happened to your body during puberty? The surge of estrogen awakened the fat cells in your breasts, buttocks, hips, and thighs—and you were given a womanly, pear-shaped body. This was your fat cells' first major assignment, and they didn't want to disappoint you. They needed to store enough fat for menstruation to start, then they needed to store even more to make sure enough fat was packed away to survive a potential famine. Through thousands of years of evolution, your fat cells learned that the larger they grew during puberty, the more calories you would have on reserve to survive a famine, drought, or other catastrophe. And just in case you were pregnant when this pending famine hit, their goal was to make sure both you *and* your developing child were protected.

Then, if and when you actually did get pregnant, high estrogen levels brought the power of your fat cells to new heights. During the entire nine months of pregnancy, your fat cells were busy storing as much fat as possible to further protect and cushion the fetus. And after you delivered your child, your fat cells were congratulating themselves for a job well done.

We have all gone through the first stage of fat storage with puberty, many of us have gone through the second stage with pregnancy (some for repeated encores), and all of us will go through the third stage with menopause. But the process is markedly different. **A surge in estrogen doesn't cause more weight gain; a drop in estrogen does.**

During menopause, many women come to the conclusion that they should be losing weight because they no longer need all that extra fat for fertility and pregnancy. When that feared famine hits, they need only enough stored fat for one person to survive, not potentially two.

Their rationale makes sense: If estrogen stimulates fat storage, then the decreased estrogen levels during perimenopause should cause weight loss, not weight gain. One would think. But the midlife fat cell is so resourceful that it finds other reasons and other ways to store fat. Now that you are a bit older, your fat cells want to make sure that you not only survive, but also live a long, healthy life. They are worried that a disease or disability may strike in the upcoming years that causes substantial weight loss and weakness. Even more important, they are concerned with your quality of life today. An amazing phenomenon occurs during menopause: To smooth your transition, balance your body, stabilize your moods, and enhance your well-being, **your fat cells grow larger to start producing estrogen for you**.

To fulfill this life-enhancing duty, they quickly activate more of the enzymes that store fat, deactivate the enzymes that release it, and expand by at least 20 percent. If you were to look at a female fat cell under the microscope, this is what it would look like before and during the transition to menopause:

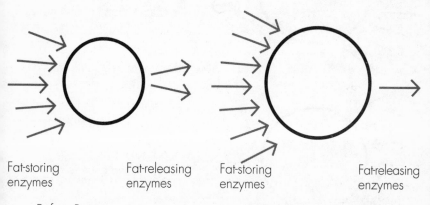

| Fat-storing enzymes | Fat-releasing enzymes | Fat-storing enzymes | Fat-releasing enzymes |

Before Perimenopause   During Perimenopause

(The arrows in this and all diagrams illustrate the enzymes that store and release fat. They do not reflect the exact number of enzymes; they are to help you visualize how female fat cells function.)

In summary, this is the healthy and necessary life cycle of a female fat cell:

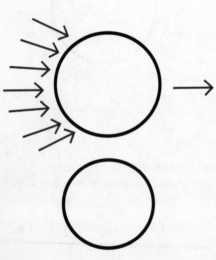

Birth – happy to be alive

Childhood – waiting patiently for puberty

Puberty – hooray!! – life is grand

Pregnancy – nine months of fat-storing celebration

Menopausal transition – wow, this is like my second puberty, only better

Postmenopause – now I can relax and enjoy my healthy, long life

Your premenopausal fat cells may have been smart and stubborn, but your menopausal fat cells are ingenious. It's their last chance to get as big and plump as they possibly can. I can't predict exactly when the IQ of your fat cells will skyrocket and you'll enter this transition or exactly how powerful and big your fat cells will become. We are all different. But what I do know is that the transition starts in your mid to late 30s, gains force through your 40s, and tapers off in your mid to late 50s. We all follow a similar timeline.

WHEN FAT CELLS TURN 35

Somewhere in your mid to late 30s, you did or will become aware of some subtle changes in your body. Your periods still come like clockwork, you are still fertile and in your childbearing years, and your hormones are still within normal ranges—but something's definitely different. You begin to notice initial changes that will continue to intensify over the next few years.

- Your partner starts identifying that you're having PMS before you do, and your premenstrual time is longer—meaning that almost half of your waking days are PMS. When you think about it, it seems like you are always either cranky or crampy.

- You are craving more chocolate, sugar, and fat—especially premenstrually.

- Your weight is starting to climb, and your morning weigh-in becomes more important than your morning coffee.

- Your waist measurement increases by at least an inch.

- You start staring in the mirror, taking inventory of changes in your body. You're positive that there's more cellulite today than there was yesterday.

- You notice that your breasts are growing, and when you turn around, you realize that it's not just your breasts, you have more fat on your back, too.

- The old standby diet that used to guarantee a five-pound weight loss in a month doesn't work anymore, and you start browsing the diet section of bookstores.

Research has finally surfaced to explain why you and your fat cells undergo such a remarkable change during "the change." *Simply stated: female fat cells can tell time, they are experts in geography, and they have a built-in laboratory to produce estrogen.*

When fat cells first detect a slightly lower estrogen level, they rise to the occasion. One fat cell says to the other, "See, I told you so. I've been counting the years and monitoring her estrogen level. She really needs our help now—wake up, recruit the extra forces, spread the word." So while your fat cells are spreading the word, you're observing the first signs of middle-age spread.

All of your other cells don't know what to do to help; they can't grow and produce estrogen on command. But your fat cells know exactly what to do: activate more fat storage enzymes and increase their size so that they will be able to produce estrogen. As your ovaries and other glands and organs start to decrease their release of estrogen, suddenly, the only reliable source of estrogen comes from your fat cells. The bigger they become, the more estrogen they will be able to produce. The University of Pittsburgh found that those women with the largest fat cells produce 40 percent more estrogen than those with the smallest ones. To become bigger and better, from the mid 30s on, the average woman puts on an additional one-and-a-half pounds of fat a year. The first pound or so will go unnoticed, but as the fat accumulates, you'll no doubt have to face the fact that your wardrobe isn't getting smaller—you're getting bigger.

This process explains why you are gaining weight without a change in your eating or exercise habits, but why are you gaining most of that annual pound and a half of fat in your waist? Because the geographical location of your abdominal fat cells is most conducive to producing estrogen. These fat cells surround the liver and adrenal glands, which lend a helping hand to produce estrogen. The adrenal glands produce a form of testosterone, the liver produces the enzyme necessary to convert the testosterone to estrogen, and the fat cells surrounding the liver and adrenal glands provide the laboratory to get the job done. It's a highly efficient system.

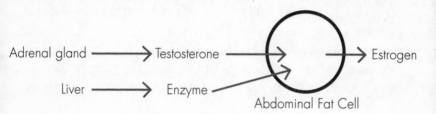

A year ago or ten years ago (depending on your age), you were more likely to store fat in your buttocks, hips, and thighs. Today, it's most likely to be in your stomach and waist. Your thighs have done their job, now it's time to rest. And while they are recuperating from years of hard work, they relax a bit too much and lose some of their structure, collapsing in certain areas and plumping out in others. Cellulite starts to become more noticeable and is often described as "dimples on your fat cells." Could it be that your thirtysomething fat cells are so happy to be in midlife that they are smiling at you?

It wouldn't surprise me. This is their heyday, and they are also ecstatic about your loss of muscle mass. Muscle loss works in tandem with fat gain. Muscle is your metabolism, and when you lose muscle, you lose your ability to burn calories. So from age 35 on, the average woman loses about a half pound of muscle a year while she's gaining one-and-a-half pounds of fat. When you lose a half pound of muscle, you burn about forty fewer calories a day. The more muscle you lose, the fewer calories your body needs, and the extra calories are rerouted to your fat cells to store.

In addition to muscle loss, food cravings also join in to give fat cells a helping hand. A slight decrease in estrogen and progesterone intensifies your PMS, mood changes, and food cravings. When estrogen levels diminish, the levels of certain brain chemicals follow suit. One of the most influential is serotonin. When serotonin levels drop below normal, you feel tired, moody, and your brain cells cry out for sugar, starch, and chocolate as a natural way to bring this important brain chemical back into balance and make you feel better. In addition, the ice cream, hot fudge, and whipped cream also help to make your fat cells feel better. Your cravings for high-calorie foods ensure that you are eating sufficient calories for your fat cells to store. During perimenopause, *everything* seems to work in the fat cells' favor.

From the combination of lower estrogen levels, less muscle mass, increased food cravings, and increased fat storage enzymes, this is what your 35-year-old fat cells look like:

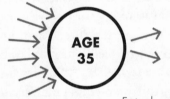

Fat-storing enzymes   Fat-releasing enzymes

When you were in your 20s, you may have cursed your female fat cells, but with the right approach to eating and exercising, you did see results. But by the time you celebrate your 40th birthday, you may have had a child or two, you are clinical evidence that gravity does exist, your waist is no longer the size of Scarlett O'Hara's—and you've lost two-and-one-half pounds of muscle, gained seven-and-one-half pounds of fat, and need 200 fewer calories a day.

With each subsequent birthday, your fat cells are having more of a celebration with the cake and ice cream than you are.

WHEN FAT CELLS TURN 45

When you reach your mid 40s, your estrogen levels are declining more significantly, your body changes are no longer subtle, and there is no question in your mind that you are in perimenopause.

- Your periods have changed—sometimes longer, other times shorter; sometimes heavier, other times lighter.

- You are craving chocolate all month long and keeping chocolate everywhere—in your purse, briefcase, desk drawer, and anywhere else that's feasible. You may be forgetting people's names and appointment times, but chocolate is excluded from your memory loss.

- You continue to lose one-half pound of muscle a year, and your caloric needs drop by as much as 400 calories a day. If you are eating the same amount, you are storing most of those 400 calories in your waist.

- You have gained up to ten pounds of fat and are more frustrated with your weight than ever before.

- One-size-fits-all labels have crept into your closet along with elastic-waisted pants and skirts.

- You are considering liposuction or any other procedure to get rid of this unwanted fat.

- Your fat cells start reproducing and multiplying to make sure there is plenty of room to store fat and produce the estrogen you need. In other words, you may not be able to give birth any longer, but your fat cells still can.

Fat cells giving birth? Many women aren't happy to hear that their fat cells are reproducing, but it's another one of their

highly evolved functions during perimenopause. Because your
ovaries' output of estrogen is now below normal, fat cells start
dividing as a safeguard for estrogen production. Their new
motto is *divide and conquer*.

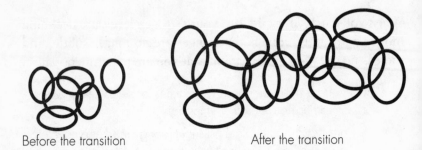

Before the transition   After the transition

When you are in your mid to late 40s, your menopausal fat
cells are working together like an ant colony, some dividing, others expanding, and all managing to store unbelievable amounts
of calories in their microscopic containers. All of this hard work
is to make sure you are gaining ample weight in your waist so
that your abdominal fat cells can provide a natural source of estrogen.

By now, your fat cells have been so successful in stimulating weight gain in your upper body that a change in body
shape is apparent. Your waist has increased two inches, and
your pear-shaped body has become noticeably more apple-
shaped. This shift in body shape is pleasing to some women.
It was to my friend Stephanie. After being pear-shaped since
puberty and having to buy smaller-size tops than bottoms for
the past thirty years, she welcomed a more even weight distribution. She came walking out of a room one day modeling
her new apple-shaped body for appraisal and asked, "What
do you think? Red delicious or Granny Smith?" We all agreed
she was red delicious—and proud of it.

This is what Stephanie's and your 45-year-old fat cells look like:

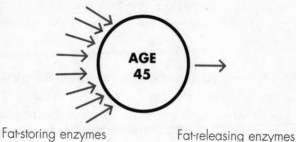

Fat-storing enzymes   Fat-releasing enzymes

As you approach the 50-year mark, your body and fat cells continue to change, and you are reading everything that you can get your hands on about menopause. It becomes the number one topic of conversation with your friends and the number one concern with your doctor. Then as you round your fifth decade, your fat cells reach a new equilibrium. Their job is done.

WHEN FAT CELLS TURN 55

When you celebrate your 55th birthday, you'll most likely fit the clinical definition of postmenopause: no periods for at least a year. This is a relief for most women, and it's a sign that the transition is coming to a close. In addition, you'll also be relieved by other positive changes that mark the end of your perimenopausal years.

- Your moods even out. Your son is no longer murmuring under his breath "mean-o-pause."

- Your memory is making a comeback. You actually remember your daughter-in-law's name again.

- You may still have a few hot flashes, but they no longer keep you awake all night or drench you in business meetings. Your emergency portable fan is no longer necessary.

- Your weight has stabilized on its own, and you are pleasantly surprised to find that you've lost a couple of pounds without really trying.

Finally some good news! Once you stop menstruating and become postmenopausal, your fat cells have successfully accomplished their mission. The storage enzymes deactivate, some of the fat-releasing enzymes get their jobs back, and your fat cells actually shrink a bit in size.

Researchers at the University of Gothenburg in Sweden found that when postmenopausal women lost weight, virtually all of their 30 billion fat cells got smaller. The fat cells in their stomachs, abdomens, thighs, and buttocks all gave up their stubborn nature and all surrendered fat.

When you were premenopausal, the fat in your buttocks, hips, and thighs was the most stubborn because it was needed for fertility and pregnancy. When you were a perimenopausal woman, the fat in your waist was the most resistant because it was needed to start producing estrogen. Now that you are postmenopausal, the fat in all areas of your body becomes a bit more amenable to giving up fat. One client asked, "You mean I have to wait until my 55th birthday to lose weight?" Absolutely not. The program offered in this book is designed to encourage weight loss *during* the menopausal transition. It's simply an added bonus that fat cells will shrink on their own after the transition.

There's more good news: You'll start noticing more cravings for protein and vegetables instead of sugar and fat. Your body is more interested in amino acids to maintain muscle mass and nutrients to keep you healthy than fat and sugar to keep your fat cells storing.

This is what your 55-year-old fat cells look like:

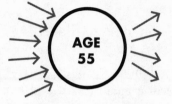

Fat-storing enzymes   Fat-releasing enzymes

Let's summarize the entire transition: Somewhere around age 35, an alarm went off in your fat cells. A slightly lower estrogen reading was detected, and your fat cells entered the transition to menopause. They knew your body's geography like the back of their hand and knew where they were needed the most. On cue, the fat cells surrounding your liver and adrenal glands were activated because this was the exact geographic location where all the necessary factors were present to produce estrogen. Then, for the rest of your transition, a convergence of factors guaranteed that you gained some extra body fat, especially in your waist.

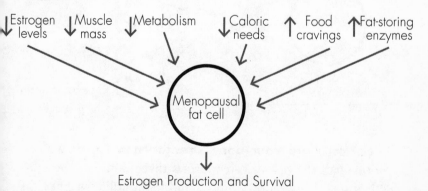

Estrogen Production and Survival

Through checks and balances and back-up plans, your fat cells made sure that they accomplished their goals of estrogen production and survival. Your health, vitality, and longevity depended on it.

FAT CELLS ARE YOUR MENOPAUSAL HELPER

With their amazing ability to produce estrogen, your fat cells provide some protection against skin and hair changes, mood swings, memory loss, fatigue, osteoporosis, and hot flashes. Every single cell in your body has receptors for estrogen. They all are affected by the decline in estrogen during perimenopause, and they all benefit from the release of estrogen once your fat cells get big enough to manufacture it. With over three hundred different functions, estrogen is not just for fertility and menstruation in your premenopausal years—it's also for your brain, bones, skin, heart, and all other organs throughout all your years.

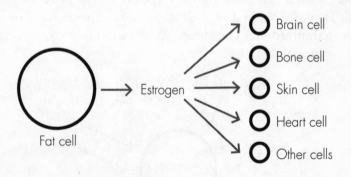

Fat cells are your bone strengthener. Larger women have one-half the risk of osteoporosis that thinner women do. The National Institute on Aging found that midlife weight gain protects against hip fractures. With the extra estrogen produced and the extra weight their skeleton had to carry around, women's hip bones became stronger and more dense. As you gain some weight during midlife, all of your bones will become stronger because simply moving your body around every day becomes weight-bearing exercise.

Fat cells are your sleep enhancer. Those who gain the most body fat during menopause have the least difficulty falling asleep. One study found that leaner women take an average of twenty-four minutes to enter the first stage of sleep while heavier women take only eleven minutes.

Fat cells are your air-conditioning. Leaner women report 50 percent more hot flashes than those who carry some additional fat. The estrogen produced by your fat cells will cool your hot flashes and night sweats.

Fat cells are your skin softener. Women who gain weight during midlife are more likely to maintain their skin collagen and natural oil production. With more fat underneath the skin, they also retain more moisture and have diminished lines and wrinkles. The anti-aging result: Larger fat cells help to slow down the skin deterioration that occurs with aging.

Fat cells really are looking out for your mental and physical well-being. But after hearing about the compelling benefits of larger fat cells, a particular question may be haunting you: "If menopausal weight gain is so healthy for me, then why is everyone saying that it's so unhealthy for me to gain weight?"

"Everyone" is not saying that, and those who do are reevaluating their positions. Midlife weight gain is not the grim reaper once thought, and thinness is not the fountain of youth once imagined.

To the contrary, fitness, not thinness, is the number one indicator of longevity. Research at The Cooper Institute for Aerobics Research in Texas has shown that thin people who are out of shape are three times more likely to die prematurely than heavier people who are in shape.

So, being thin appears to offer little protection against early death. But what about other past studies finding that thinner people have a lower disease risk and live longer? None of them factored in fitness. And except for one highly publicized study, all others have demonstrated that the health risks for carrying extra weight are much lower for women than for men.

That highly publicized study I'm referring to was conducted at Harvard a few years back, and I'm sure you remember the attention it received. We were informed that a 35-year-old woman who is 5 feet 5 inches tall should weigh in at 119 pounds. If she weighed 120 to 149, her chances of an early death rose 20 percent. If she weighed more than 150, her chances rose to 30 percent.

All of a sudden, I found myself in an earlier death category. And, all of a sudden, I was flooded with phone calls. Women who were just starting to feel good about themselves at 140 or 150 pounds were once again weight and food preoccupied—and thinking about dieting.

Before you let that negative thought enter your mind, let's do a reality check. This Harvard study was done on nurses, who represent one of the most stressed professions (and stress affects our health and our weight), it didn't control for body fat, and it didn't factor in fitness. Even without these pitfalls, the most important reality is, for most of us, that the only chance of seeing 119 pounds again is by flipping through old photo albums.

Here is some additional proof that thin may not be better:

- Cornell University researchers analyzed sixty studies from around the world involving 357,000 men and 249,000 women and found that being moderately overweight did not increase mortality. Actually, what they did find is that both extremes of underweight and overweight increased mortality, but for everyone in between, weight was not a risk factor.

- Researchers at Stanford University found that the larger a woman's thighs, the lower her risk of heart disease—especially if she also has a larger waist. Fat cells in the waist can deliver fat to the liver where it's packaged with cholesterol and released into the bloodstream. But the fat cells in the thighs just store fat; they take fat out of our system and keep it there, saving it for that pending famine. So, thin thighs don't offer the protection against heart disease that thicker thighs do—and thigh fat is only detrimental to our egos.

- Even if a woman is apple-shaped and carries a great deal of weight in her upper body, her risk of heart disease is not as high as a man's because her abdominal fat cells aren't as active. Research has found that a woman's abdominal fat cells are so busy producing estrogen that they don't release as many fatty acids to the liver to form cholesterol.

- The National Institute on Aging found that those people who lived the longest gained a moderate amount of weight in midlife. Those who gained a lot of weight *or* lost a lot of weight died younger.

Some midlife weight gain is healthy—and fitness, not thinness, is the key to a long life. Of course, you don't want to gain too much weight and increase your risk of heart disease, cancer, diabetes, and other weight-related diseases. You don't want to gain so much weight that it compromises your ability to move, play, dance, and enjoy life. When does some weight gain become too much?

On an individual level, that's a difficult question to answer because each of us is biologically unique. What may be a healthy weight gain for me may be too much for you, or vice versa. But on a grander scale, studies have found that gaining up to ten pounds during midlife is considered perfectly acceptable. As we tip the scales significantly above that, health and mobility may start to deteriorate. And if we gain thirty plus pounds, our risk of breast cancer and heart disease can double.

For the majority of us, menopause alone won't cause this kind of excessive weight gain. However, overeating and under-exercising during our menopausal years can certainly be the culprit. Our sedentary lifestyle is to blame for the rise in obesity over the last few decades, not our midlife transition. Menopause may naturally cause a five- or ten- or fifteen-pound gain, depending on your individual physiology. But as long as you're fit, this amount of weight gain will not increase your risk of disease and may be a whole lot healthier for you in the long run.

Women can gain some weight in midlife and still be healthy. We can carry some fat in our waists and still be healthy. Our bodies are designed to store fat throughout life, and we live longer with an extra reserve of calories. Finally, a medical fact that favors women and puts men at a disadvantage.

TAKING THE MEN OUT OF MENOPAUSE

When it comes to fat cells, life transitions, weight loss, and weight gain, there is no such thing as equality of the sexes.

Actually, men's fat cells have a fairly boring existence. At puberty, young men gain muscle and lose fat. And of course, men don't experience the fat-storing frenzy of pregnancy or menopause. Steady testosterone levels keep men's fat cells smaller with more releasing enzymes and fewer storage enzymes.

When researchers analyzed a fat cell from a man's buttocks and one from a woman's buttocks, this is what they found:

- a woman's fat cell is five times larger than a man's
- a woman's fat cell has more than twice the fat-storing enzymes
- a woman's fat cell has half the fat-releasing enzymes

The weight battle of the sexes continues. Men also carry about forty pounds more muscle on their bodies, and therefore, have faster metabolisms. Because of these factors, men can eat 30 percent more calories than we can (without gaining weight) and can burn 30 percent more calories during aerobic exercise than we can. They even burn more calories while sleeping—about 200 calories more. So whether they're eating, exercising, or snoring, they are disposing of calories with little effort.

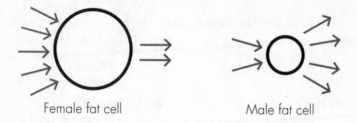

Female fat cell   Male fat cell

No wonder men have more success with dieting: they lose twice as much weight, twice as quickly, and are twice as likely to keep it off as we are. By virtue of their gender, they have the fat-burning machinery to lose weight quickly and efficiently. But they are also cast into this world with a relative inability to survive a famine. Anthropological studies have found that up to 50 percent of men perished in famines, while only 10 percent of us did. We can thank estrogen and menopause for our antifamine protection.

As men grow older, they do lose some muscle mass, but we lose twice as much. They do gain some body fat, but we gain twice as much. Weight gain peaks for men at age 44, for us at age 55 (right as we're exiting the transition to menopause). Somewhere around age 40, men experience a slow decline in testosterone, but for the next thirty years, their levels are still within the "normal" ranges. In comparison, between the ages of 35 and 55, we experience a 75 percent drop in estrogen.

I often wonder what would happen if men encountered the fat-storing effects of estrogen and menopause. What would their bodies go through and how would they cope with it? One interesting study attempted to explore this question by injecting men with estrogen. Within days they gained weight—and it took months to lose it!

Perhaps all men need to be injected with estrogen just once so they can have a hands-on understanding of what women struggle with. In lieu of estrogen injections or dissolving birth control pills in their beverages, share the following table with the men in your life and give them a crash course on the gender differences in fat cells.

MEN HAVE:

30 billion fat cells

smaller fat cells

more fat-releasing enzymes

the ability to lose weight quickly

greater success with dieting

greater success with exercise

more muscle mass (forty pounds more)

faster metabolisms (30 percent faster)

less muscle loss with age

testosterone and a shorter lifespan

fat cells that look like this:

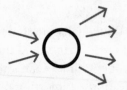

WOMEN HAVE:

30 billion smart, stubborn fat cells

larger fat cells (five times larger!)

more fat-storing enzymes

the ability to gain weight quickly

a resistance to dieting

a resistance to exercise

more fat mass

slower metabolisms

more weight gain with age

estrogen, the life-giving functions of pregnancy and breast-feeding, and a longer lifespan

fat cells that look like this:

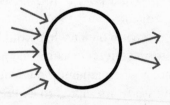

After Sheila shared this information with her husband, they concluded, "Our fat cells are worlds apart. Maybe men's fat cells really are from Mars and women's are from Venus." Maybe so, but this isn't to say that some men don't struggle with their weights. Gender is one side of the weight-gain story, genetics is the other, and lifestyle is involved in both. But we have a biological explanation for our midlife weight gain; they don't. We also have a biological advantage for living longer that they haven't figured out yet.

When it comes to longevity, Mother Nature definitely favors her own gender. Of children born today, one in three girls will live to be one hundred years old, but only one in ten boys will. Of those alive today, women will outlive men by eight years, and men are more likely to die earlier from just about every cause of death. Our bodies and fat cells are doing something right. Men lose twice as much weight as they grow older. From age 60 on, they lose twenty-eight pounds, we only lose fourteen. Our ability to hold on to fat gives us the ability to hold on to life.

I hope that you now understand the necessity of midlife weight gain and realize that *you* are not gaining weight, *your body* is. And your body is dedicated to this weight gain for essential reasons. Having this knowledge is vital, and it doesn't mean that you can't do anything about it. You may not be able to prevent menopausal body changes entirely, but with the guidance in this book, you can minimize them, shrink your fat cells without compromising their ability to produce estrogen, and find a new healthy weight that's right for you and your body.

As in puberty and pregnancy, all women *need* to gain *some* weight during menopause. Gaining too much *or* too little can compromise our health and well-being. Can you see your doctor monitoring your weight gain in menopause as in pregnancy? "Oh good! You've gained three pounds; you're right on target."

Or, "You're in your third year of perimenopause and have only gained one pound—better focus on gaining weight."

This kind of menopausal care may seem preposterous today, but as society gains a greater understanding of why women need to gain some weight during midlife, it may very well happen in the future.

chapter two

WHAT TYPE OF MIDLIFE FAT CELLS DO YOU HAVE?

All women go through menopause and all women have stubborn, efficient midlife fat cells. These are medical facts that we must accept and work with. But before you start making positive lifestyle changes to keep midlife weight gain to a minimum, it's important to get acquainted with the specifics of *your* fat cells and tailor the information on menopausal physiology to your personal situation. **The more you know about your fat cells, the more successful you'll be in outsmarting them.**

No two women have the same menopausal experience, and no two women have the exact same changes in body shape, weight, fat cells, and metabolism. All you need to do is get a group of women together and ask a few personal midlife questions to get hundreds of different answers—which is exactly what I did.

- To the question: **How much weight have you gained?**, the answers spanned from two unnoticeable pounds to fifty-two unbelievable ones. Some women gained the majority of their weight at the beginning of the transition, others toward the end, and still others steadily throughout.

- To the question: **How has your figure changed?**, the answers ranged from "losing it completely along with my libido" to "everyone says I look the same, but I don't believe them."

- To the question: **How would you describe the intensity of your experience?**, the answers ranged from mild to moderate to massive—with most leaning toward the massive changes.

- To the question: **How does your experience compare with your mother's?**, the answers varied from a handful saying "exactly the same" to most reporting "there is no comparison."

If you look to your mother's perimenopausal experience for a sense of what's to come, most of you will find few similarities to your own. Her transition averaged six months to three years; yours will be ten to twenty years. She may have experienced weight gain, hot flashes, mood swings, memory loss, and insomnia too, but nowhere near the degree you are. She gained eight pounds compared to your twelve and reported three hot flashes a day to your fifteen.

Over the past few decades, there has been an amazing demographic shift for menopause. It no longer starts in the late 40s, but in the late 30s. It doesn't last a couple of years; it lasts more than a decade. It doesn't produce mild changes; it causes megamenopausal changes.

What makes our generation so different?

In the same group of women I surveyed on midlife body changes, I asked this very question. Before you read on, think about how you might explain this menopausal shift.

One group member said, "I think it's because more of us have decided not to have children." Another immediately interjected, "You're right, and even when we do have children, we're having fewer, later in life."

This is true and explains at least part of the difference. Each full-term pregnancy pushes off menopause by five months. So if your mother had five children, her transition began twenty-five months later, and this explains about two years of the difference.

A third group member said, "I think it's because we've taken birth control pills for years, some since our teens." To my knowledge, the effect of long term oral contraceptive use on menopause has never been studied, but a theory has been proposed. Taking the pill for years may cause our bodies to become dependent on an external source of hormones and, therefore, our ovaries get lazy and produce less estrogen over time. Thus, earlier perimenopause.

Another woman asked, "Could it be because we started puberty earlier? And if so, what does this mean for my daughter? She started her period a year before I did." The relationship between age at puberty and age at perimenopause has been studied, and there appears to be a correlation. We entered puberty at an earlier age than our mothers did, and we're entering the transition at a much earlier age. As for our daughters' generation, only time will tell.

Then a determined woman took the floor, "I know why our generation is so different. It's because we're too stressed, and stress affects everything, so it must affect menopause. My mother didn't have a career outside of the home, she didn't commute three hours a day, and she didn't have to worry as much about gangs, drive-by shootings, teen pregnancy, drugs, and AIDS."

Stress, although difficult to study because it's so subjective, has been linked to an earlier menopause. When we are under chronic stress, the adrenal glands are constantly releasing cortisol, and this competes with their ability to release testosterone, the precursor to estrogen.

When I asked, "What else have we been doing that adds an immense amount of stress to our bodies and lives?" everyone drew a blank.

The answer is *dieting*.

Dieting is both a physiological and psychological stress and may be the most influential factor for our longer transition and megamenopausal experience. It triggers a release of stress hormones, preoccupies our minds, and causes feelings of guilt when we eat and depression when we don't reach our goals. Everything about dieting is stressful: undereating, overexercising, bingeing, skipping meals, and taking diet pills. Studies have shown that undernourished women enter menopause four years earlier than those who eat an adequate amount of calories for their bodies.

Half of us started undernourishing our bodies as teenagers and most of the rest of us joined in by the time we reached 25. Our mothers came of age when thinness wasn't a primary goal and dieting was not an American pastime. Their bodies were better nourished and in a better balance to help them through the transition. We are coming of age when thinness and dieting are obsessions, and our bodies are out of balance long before we enter perimenopause.

Depending on your mother's age, this generational analysis may be better suited for comparing and contrasting your grandmother's experience. If you are 35 years old and your mother is 55, she's at the tail end of the transition and, as a younger woman, was very much affected by the same contemporary issues with stress, dieting practices, and reproductive choices as you have been.

Let's move this discussion from your mother (or your grandmother) to you: How much weight have you gained? How has your body shape changed? What factors do you think are responsible for magnifying your changes?

One of my clients answered, "I've gained twenty-three pounds since my late 30s, my hourglass figure ran out years ago, and I think I have every factor working against me to cause massive body changes. I started dieting when I was 11 years old and have yo-yoed too many times to count. I started the Pill at age 18, had one child at age 38, and stress is the first thing I feel when I get up in the morning and the last thing I feel when I can't fall asleep at night. No wonder I've gained twenty-three pounds!"

The amount of weight you gain and where you gain it depends on your current and past lifestyle, dieting practices, medical history, hormone use, and to some extent, genetics. Circle all those factors that are influencing or have influenced the power and efficiency of your midlife fat cells.

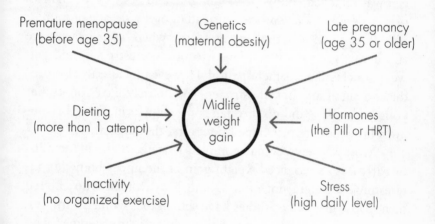

For those variables that you can't control such as premature menopause, genetics, and late pregnancy, it's important to acknowledge their influence for a better understanding of how your body is traveling through menopause. For those you can control such as stress, inactivity, dieting, and other eating habits, it's not only important to understand their past influence, but also to take future action. This chapter will continue to build on your understanding of midlife fat cells, and the remainder of this book will give you the skills to outsmart them.

FAT CELLS PREMATURELY FORCED INTO MENOPAUSE

If you've had a complete hysterectomy (where your ovaries as well as your uterus were surgically removed) or had chemotherapy or radiation, or were on a particular drug that interfered with your sex hormones, your body was forced into premature menopause. You experienced many of the same changes as women who undergo natural menopause except that it wasn't a transition; it was an abrupt loss of female hormones. Your primary source of estrogen was removed, and your weight gain and body shape changes occurred within a few months instead of over a decade or more.

If you had a partial hysterectomy where your ovaries are still intact, your body continued to produce estrogen, and you were not classified as menopausal. However, the uterus also produces a small amount of estrogen, so you may have found that your body shape did go through some transformations, becoming a little more apple-shaped right after the surgery.

Most women who had complete hysterectomies in their 20s or early 30s experienced weight gain in the upper body, but interestingly enough, not quite as much as women who entered menopause naturally. Studies have shown that women with hysterectomies gained about one-half of the weight of women who had natural menopause. Why? At least part of the answer is that fat cells follow a general timeline. They were not programmed to enter menopause or to expand in size and number at age 30.

That's why even though you had a hysterectomy years ago, you'll most likely go through a type of menopausal transition again. As you reach the time in your life where you would naturally have stopped menstruating, you'll notice your body changing, your moods changing, and your sleep patterns changing—for the second time. Your fat cells follow their prime directive, and you'll gain the rest of your weight then and go through the rest of your transition.

POSTPARTUM FAT CELLS ENTERING MENOPAUSE WHILE BREAST-FEEDING

This is as complicated as it sounds.

Because women are waiting longer to have children, an "over 40" pregnancy, almost unheard of in our mothers' generation, is now becoming quite common. If you get pregnant at the beginning of the transition, estrogen levels soar instead of drop, and the fat cells in your buttocks, hips, and thighs put on an extra ten pounds. Then, after you deliver your child, estrogen levels drop because you're postpartum—and continue dropping because you are entering menopause.

We don't know where pregnancy weight gain ends and menopausal weight gain begins. We don't know when postpartum depression ends and menopausal mood changes begin. Because of these blurred boundaries, many women, like Sally, are confused during this time. "I always knew that there was something more to my postpartum depression. It never went away. My midwife said it was the 'baby blues' and would disappear within a couple of weeks. But two years later, I feel like nothing has disappeared—including my pregnancy weight. "

Women don't have the time to lose the weight they gained during pregnancy before their fat cells realize that they are in perimenopause and want to multiply and store again for different reasons. Two of the most powerful fat-storing times in a woman's life are occurring simultaneously. And if a third factor, breast-feeding, is added to this scenario, fat cells want to hold on to their fat for dear life—just in case that famine hits while your infant is dependent on your milk production for survival. Even though we read and are told that breast-feeding leads to weight loss, most women report that they don't lose weight until after they stop breast-feeding. If pregnancy and breast-feeding are a part of your midlife weight gain experience, look on the positive side. You have a new child to go along with any extra weight. Most women are thankful to conceive later in life and grateful to know the reasons why they are gaining weight (instead of losing) in the years following delivery.

GENETICALLY OVERACTIVE FAT CELLS

If larger fat cells run in your family, expect more weight gain during the transition. The more you weigh as you enter menopause, the more you'll weigh by the time it's over.

Some of my clients think this makes no sense at all. "I already have more than enough stored fat to produce the estrogen my body needs, so why on earth would my body want to store more?" Because the female body seems to want to gain a proportionate amount of fat during the transition. In chapter 1, you learned that midlife fat cells increase their size by about 20 percent during the transition. No matter if they are small, medium, or large at the onset of your perimenopausal years, they are programmed to grow 20 percent larger. One study found that overweight women gained an average of twenty-two pounds during perimenopause, while women at a more comfortable weight gained twelve pounds.

How do you know if you have genetically overactive fat cells? Laura asked this question, and we explored her lifestyle and family history for the answer. Her 5 foot 9 inch body was the mirror image of her mother's. They both had large bones, large breasts, and large thighs, and gained a large amount of weight (twenty-five pounds) during the transition. Both Laura and her mother exercised, didn't overeat, and didn't diet. This was where Laura's body genetically felt the most comfortable. Her lifestyle was not responsible; her genetically overactive fat cells were.

FAT CELLS ON HORMONES

If you are on the Pill or on hormone replacement therapy (HRT), another variable is added to the mystery of midlife weight gain.

Some women are on birth control pills to prevent pregnancy or add a little extra estrogen during the transition (the Pill is sometimes recommended before HRT). That little extra estrogen can cause a 1 to 2 percent increase in body fat. If you've been on the Pill for years, you've already gained the fat associated with its use. But, if you've just started oral contraceptives, you can expect some increased fat in the buttocks, hips, and thighs.

With HRT, the dose is higher than the Pill, and the extra estrogen can cause even more storage in the lower body. Some studies have found that women on HRT gain more weight and body fat; others found no significant difference in the amount of weight gained, but a difference in where it was gained. Women on HRT gained more fat in the lower body because estrogen feeds the fat cells of the buttocks, hips, and thighs. In fact, a group of European researchers found that thigh storage increased by 50 percent with HRT. This may not sound desirable to you, but larger thighs may be one of the reasons why HRT reduces the risk of heart disease. Being pear-shaped is good for the heart.

As one woman surmised, "I gained weight in the waist when I started the transition, then I went on HRT and I gained weight in the thighs. Now I have more fat everywhere!"

This woman also asked if going off HRT would lead to weight loss. Discontinuing hormone replacement might trigger some weight loss in the lower body, but it is beyond my realm of expertise to advise for or against HRT. We need to weigh the risks against the benefits, discuss the options with our physician, and if we determine that our bodies need hormone replacement to improve our quality of life, then any weight gain in the thighs will have to be accepted as part of the package.

UNFIT FAT CELLS UNDER STRESS

Women are under more stress than ever before in history. According to the United Nations Report on the Status of Women, we do two-thirds of the world's work for one-tenth of the world's wages. We are so stressed doing the work of the world that we don't have enough time to exercise. Not a good combination. Other than removing stress from your life (a seemingly impossible feat), exercise is the most effective way to tame your body's response to stress.

During the fight or flight response, a release of adrenaline, cortisol, and other stress hormones causes a cascade of reactions to increase your chances of survival—to fight for your life or to flee as fast as you possibly can. The problem with many of the sources of contemporary stress is that fighting or fleeing is unrealistic. You cannot necessarily knock out your boss or run away from a deadline. I guess you could, but then you'd have to deal with the stress of lawsuits and unemployment.

So the stress of day-to-day life keeps building, the stress hormones keep accumulating, and you keep gaining weight. Stress causes additional menopausal weight gain in three ways:

1. **Increased fat storage.** Stress threatens your fat cells and stimulates more fat-storage enzymes in response to the potentially life-threatening situation. But stress is selective in which fat cells it activates: The thigh area is ignored while the abdominal area is targeted because these fat cells can more easily come to your aid with a burst of energy to save your life.

2. **Decreased estrogen production.** From years of stress, your adrenal glands have been so busy producing the stress hormones that they are too worn out to produce the needed testosterone to make estrogen in your fat cells. To offset lower estrogen levels, the fat cells in your waist grow bigger and bigger to try to get the job done.

3. **Increased stress eating.** During the period of recovery from stress, your appetite center is stimulated, causing you to eat more calories. Stress eating is not just for emotional reasons; it's also for physiological ones. And when you do eat, the fat-storage enzymes are ready and waiting to store more of the calories in your waist. Stress eating makes your fat cells quite happy.

You may know people who lose weight when they are under stress. We all react differently to major life events and anxiety-producing situations. A few report decreased appetite with stress, but those people who lose a significant amount of weight are usually reacting to more than just commuter traffic or crying children; they may have experienced a death or other traumatic event.

You may know others who maintain their weight when they are under stress—because they're fit. If you exercise, you know what a wonderful stress release it can be and how it reduces stress eating. Physical fitness builds up our resistance to stress by metabolizing the stress hormones and helping our bodies recover. Without exercise, the accumulating stress hormones have a detrimental effect on our fat cells and menopausal experience, causing more hot flashes, insomnia, and other discomforts.

Of course, exercise does a lot more than reduce stress. It also directly reduces the size of our midlife fat cells. Aerobic exercise and strength training will be discussed and recommended in upcoming chapters, but as an early plug for fitness, let me share the motivating results of a study conducted at the Washington University School of Medicine. Fit women enter the transition carrying less body fat and gain less fat during it.

	PREMENOPAUSAL WOMEN	POSTMENOPAUSAL WOMEN
SEDENTARY	carried 32 lbs of fat	carried 59 lbs of fat
FIT	carried 21 lbs of fat	carried 33 lbs of fat

The sedentary women gained 27 pounds of fat from their pre- to postmenopausal years—that's almost two and a half times more than the fit women! No one can argue these results. **Exercise combats menopausal fat!**

FAT CELLS WITH A LONG HISTORY OF DIETING

At what age did you start dieting? How many diets have you been on? How much weight have you lost dieting? How much weight have you regained?

The earlier you started dieting and the more diets you've been on, the more weight you'll gain during the transition. An estimated one-third of the weight we gain is caused by the weight we've lost and regained with dieting. If the average weight gain during perimenopause is twelve pounds, then at least four of them can be blamed on dieting.

"So, if I never dieted, I'd be four pounds lighter right now?" Probably. You also wouldn't be thinking about another diet.

Dieting during menopause is even more detrimental than dieting before you reach menopause. It only gives your fat cells more power and speeds up the weight-gain process. You'll lose muscle faster, gain fat faster, and manufacture more fat-storage enzymes. You can't change your dieting past, but you *can* change your dieting future.

You may have been dieting all along and figure "Why stop now?" Or you may have given up dieting a few years back. Or you may have never really been a serious dieter, but all of a sudden, your diet antenna has risen. Your ears are perked for any mention of weight loss and dieting. You start staying up a bit later than usual to watch the weight-loss infomercials. Eventually, you jump out of the chair announcing, "I have to get this weight off; I'll do anything!"

If you are tempted to go on a diet, take the newest diet pill, or try the latest weight-loss craze, please read on. Dieting not only makes your midlife fat cells larger, it makes your menopausal experience worse.

You probably consider yourself a bright woman with years of wisdom and experience, but when it comes to dieting, your intelligence can take a nosedive. We believe the claims of ingenious marketers, magazine ads, and infomercials. But in reality, not much has changed for over fifty years. The first study to identify the negative effects of food restriction was conducted during World War II. The food-deprived soldiers became preoccupied with food, ate like crazy when food was finally available, and put on more weight than they had lost during the war. Even those who were genetically underweight before the war battled their weight after the war.

Since then dozens of studies have been done confirming the same results. The only difference is that instead of involuntary food restriction, the restriction was intentional. We have deprived ourselves of necessary calories, nutrients, and energy—not once, but over and over again. A *Consumer Reports* survey on almost 100,000 dieters found that those who yo-yoed the most weighed the most. As far as your fat cells are concerned, each diet has been a famine and each postdiet binge has been a feast to celebrate the end of the famine.

As soon as you go on a diet, your brain starts sending signals down nerve pathways to your fat cells to alert them that "the diet is coming, the diet is coming." Like Paul Revere and the patriots, your fat cells respond quickly to get ready for battle. When you were 12, 22, and 32 years old, the same message was sent to stimulate fat storage, but now that you're perimenopausal, the message is fast and furious. And it is sent directly to the fat cells in your abdomen. Today, your abdominal fat cells will fight back because they have the important job of producing estrogen, and no fat-burning pill, no high-protein diet, no weight-loss plan is going to get the best of them.

As a menopausal woman, you probably won't lose any weight with your next diet but may actually gain weight instead. You won't even have those few months of slender bliss before you gain the weight back; you'll skip the first phase and go straight to the weight gain.

One of my clients didn't believe a word of it. "I've always lost weight dieting. I've always gained it back too, but that's not the point. I can lose weight now, and I'll prove it to you." She marched off to a local weight-loss center where she gathered up her 800-calorie meal plans and diet pills and was instructed to come back the following Tuesday for her weekly weigh-in. A week went by, no loss. Her diet counselor told her that her body may be resisting weight loss (the only accurate piece of information she received) and to be patient until next week. She waited, not so patiently, and gained a pound. Now her counselor told her that she must not be following the meal plans or taking her diet pills. After a few minutes of arguing that she was doing everything she was supposed to be doing, she said, "I'll tell you what I'm not doing. I'm not coming back here again!"

When she called to tell me about her experience, I was sorry that she had to go through the failure and humiliation, but sometimes we need one last diet attempt to find out for ourselves. I hope that this woman's experience will help you overcome the need to prove to yourself that *diets do not work*.

You can't force your fat cells to shrink during midlife; they have to grow to produce estrogen. If you try to starve them, they'll figure out how to manipulate the situation to their advantage. They'll ask, "How can I keep storing even though she's not eating?" They'll boost their fat-storing enzymes and banish their fat-releasing enzymes. Then they'll recruit the help of your muscle mass by breaking it down and slowing down your metabolism. The combination of a slower metabolism and efficient storage makes it possible to store even the lowest-calorie foods as fat. Millions of midlife women are storing rice cakes, carrot sticks, and celery in their fat cells.

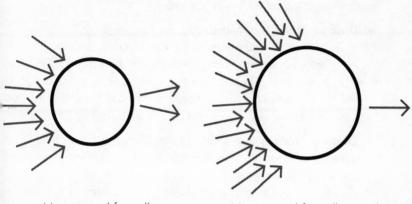

Menopausal fat cell   Menopausal fat cell on a diet

The only thing your perimenopausal fat cells haven't figured out a way to store yet is water—but I wouldn't put it past them. If we keep dieting, we may see a front page headline reporting, "Water Makes Us Fat."

In summary, fat cells become more efficient at storage during the transition to menopause, but dieting makes them super-efficient by doubling the fat-storage enzymes and cutting the fat-releasing enzymes in half.

Dieting does a lot more to your menopausal body than make your fat cells exponentially expand. Everything you've been concerned about during midlife, from memory loss to hair loss and from osteoporosis to insomnia, may be partially caused by dieting and is definitely exacerbated by dieting. A dieting perimenopausal woman experiences a faster and more significant drop in estrogen. That's why dieting thins everything—but your body.

- **Dieting thins your hair.** Dieting at any age has been linked to hair loss. But as we reach menopause, we lose hair naturally from lower estrogen levels, then we lose even more hair by dieting. One in three women is reporting significant hair thinning during the transition, making hair loss one of the fastest-growing (pardon the pun) midlife complaints.

- **Dieting thins your muscle.** You are already losing a half pound of muscle each year during the transition, and you'll lose it even faster by dieting. About 30 percent of the weight lost on low-calorie diets comes from muscle breakdown. So, if you starve yourself to lose ten pounds in a month, that's three pounds of muscle lost, and you've aged your body by six years in thirty days!

- **Dieting thins your skin.** Dieting decreases the strength of connective tissue so that your muscles don't adhere to your fat and skin like they used to, and the tissue sags. Dieting also decreases skin tone and elasticity, making lines and wrinkles more apparent. The dieting-wrinkle connection is often the motivating factor for women to stop dieting once and for all.

- **Dieting thins your bones.** Dieting makes your bones more porous and fragile, increasing the likelihood of fractures and increasing your risk of osteoporosis. With dieting, calcium intake is often lower, too, adding to the loss of bone density.

- **Dieting thins your thinking.** The recent headline "Dieting Makes You Dumb" struck me as a rather crude way of announcing research findings, but it definitely got the point across. "Diet dummies" were identified when The Institute of Food Research in England found that dieting dulled memory and decreased mental acuity within forty-eight hours.

Dieting also decreases concentration, attention span, productivity, and reaction time. It takes longer to complete tasks, figure out problems, react in an emergency, and generally get things done. Maybe dieting is the real culprit, not menopause. Our lack of mental efficiency may be caused by an excess in dieting.

A client called me up after reading about "dieting dummies" and concluded, "I may have been dumb to diet, but I'm not stupid. I'm never dieting again." She was a professor at a prestigious university and perhaps smarter than anyone I know, but this news report is what got her to stop dieting and start using her smarts to really outsmart her midlife fat cells.

You, too, can stop dieting and start using your smarts. What you've done in the past isn't as important as what you do in the future. If you haven't been consistent with exercise, if you have been consistent with dieting—*that's okay*. You have another opportunity to do something good for your body. The most important one of your life.

Even if you've been on a hundred diets, you can reverse the damage. The question is not "What have I done?"; it's *"What can I do differently now?"* You can turn the page and start taking The Meno-Positive Approach to a Trimmer Transition.

chapter three

THE MENO-POSITIVE
APPROACH TO A
TRIMMER TRANSITION

After a few months of making phone calls in hopes of finding a weight management program designed specifically for menopausal women, Michelle rang me. She began by giving me a detailed history of her weight, eating habits, and lifestyle, and explaining that she had kept her weight perfectly stable until two years ago. I sat back in my chair listening sympathetically, ready to take my turn to explain her menopausal weight gain. But Michelle immediately went into her list of ten specific questions for me to answer on my approach and philosophies.

I was impressed with her level of organization and commitment to finding a program that was right for both her life and her body. She was impressed with my honest answers and knowledge about women's health and weight loss. At the end of our conversation, she said that she thought she wanted to work with me, but had one last question: "What do you call your positive approach to helping women control their weight during menopause?" I responded, "I call it The Meno-Positive Approach to a Trimmer Transition."

Michelle loved the name of my program, but more important, she felt that this approach made complete sense from a physiological standpoint. Menopausal fat cells are undergoing enormous changes, so eating and exercise habits have to change with them.

I asked Michelle to share the list of ten questions she asked me on the phone because they may be the same questions you have, and answering them now will prepare you for The Meno-Positive Approach.

1. **What's the most important change I can make during the transition to lose weight?** Without hesitation, the answer is *exercise*. Aerobic exercise combined with strength building is the only way to stimulate the release of fat from your fat cells. During menopause, your fat cells are storing more, but the right exercise program can counteract at least half of that storage. That's why we'll first focus on tailoring your exercise program to work for menopause.

2. **How many menopausal women have you worked with?** Over two thousand at various stages of the transition. Through their experiences and my own research, I've discovered what works and what doesn't. But it's important to keep in mind that we are all different physiologically and psychologically, and the changes we make must realistically fit into our day-to-day lifestyles.

3. **What is your success rate?** One hundred percent if the measure of success is a greater understanding and acceptance of our bodies during the transition—which for me is the most important measurement. If I help you to change your attitudes and habits to enhance your body image, fitness, and well-being, then I have accomplished my primary goals. Most women, however, evaluate success by the numbers on the scale. I cannot guarantee that you'll reach your preconceived weight goal (which may not be realistic), but I can guarantee that you'll reach a healthy weight, lose your preoccupation with dieting, and gain muscle, stamina, and strength from your exercise program.

4. **How much weight can I expect to lose?** It's impossible to give you a single answer because it depends on where you are when you start the program. If you've been moderate with eating

and committed to exercise and have still gained weight, then at a minimum you'll prevent any additional weight gain and may lose a few pounds of fat. If you've already gained too much body fat because of repeated dieting and overeating, then you'll lose that excess amount—it may be five pounds or fifty pounds. Since most perimenopausal women are gaining more weight than they need to, nearly all of my clients lose some fat.

5. **How do you measure results?** Not by the scale. I don't have one in my office or in my home for that matter. Your own perceptions of body changes—such as how your clothes fit and how you feel—are most important. I do, however, recommend and use body composition analysis so that we can measure pounds of muscle gained and pounds of fat lost over time. For example, if you gain three pounds of muscle and lose three pounds of fat, the numbers on the scale won't have changed, but your body will have. It will be leaner and smaller because muscle is more compact than fat.

6. **Do you have weekly meal plans for me to follow?** No, structured meal plans work only for as long as you're following them, which is often only two weeks or a month at best. Instead, I'll help you follow your body's optimal meal plan by getting in touch with your menopausal food needs and responding to your signals of hunger and fullness.

7. **Will you have me count calories and grams of fat?** No, if counting calories and grams of fat were the secret to weight loss, your search would have been over years ago. What you eat is less important than why, when, and how much you eat.

8. **Do I have to give up any of my favorite foods?** Absolutely not! In fact, I recommend the opposite: incorporating your favorite foods into a healthy lifestyle. As you know all too well, restriction only cries out for overindulgence. *Whatever you resist, persists.* But the more satisfied you are with what you're eating, the less you'll need to eat, and the better you'll feel.

9. **Do you sell any products like fat-burning supplements or prepackaged foods?** I never have and never will. For those who do sell weight-loss products, profit is often the underlying motive.

10. **How does your approach differ from other programs?** A variety of other programs also focus on behavior change and the lifestyle approach, but I am not aware of any designed specifically for menopausal women. The Meno-Positive Approach combines education with action by recommending eating and exercise strategies that work with your changing body. With a body-centered and person-centered approach, you make the decisions based on your understanding of the facts, what makes the most sense to you, and what is most important to you.

From the first two chapters, you have the education, understanding, and facts. You know about the effects of changing hormones on your fat cells, muscle mass, body shape, and metabolism. You also know the type of fat cells you have and the factors that have influenced your weight-gain experience. Now, it's time to put that knowledge into action. It's time to outsmart your midlife fat cells.

TEACHING 35- TO 55-YEAR-OLD FAT CELLS NEW TRICKS

Whether you are just entering the transition or just completing it, whether you've been exercising for the past twenty years or have exercised only once for twenty minutes, whether you've spent your life dieting or have never dieted in your life (a handful of you do exist)—this program will help you change the physiology of your menopausal fat cells so that you will *not* gain more weight than is necessary and healthy for you.

The overall goal is to alter the way your fat cells function—so that they store a bit less and release much more. This is the only way to manage midlife weight gain permanently. *Permanently* is the operative word. The changes you make as a result of reading this book will still be ingrained ten years from now. And twenty years down the road, your fat cells will still be storing less and releasing more.

But let's focus on today first. At this very moment, you may be doing everything to encourage fat storage. You are not doing this on purpose; years of dieting and society's restrictive eating rules have caused most of us to be in a perpetual state of fat storage. You may be depriving your body of calories, restricting fat and sugar, skipping meals, overeating when you do eat, consuming the majority of your food intake at night, and avoiding exercise at all costs.

Through decades of practicing these behaviors, your fat cells know only how to store. And through the last few years of also being perimenopausal, their storage power is turned up even more, and these habits are making your fat cells larger than ever.

With The Meno-Positive Approach, you'll teach your fat cells that they can function differently by discouraging storage and encouraging the release of fat. Your fat cells expect you to diet; they are anxiously awaiting your next calorie-deprived Monday so that they can activate storage. But when you wake up Monday morning, bypass the bathroom scale and head directly into the kitchen for breakfast, your fat cells start deactivating their fat-storage enzymes. The most effective way to trick your midlife fat cells is never to diet again and eat instead—when you are hungry, frequently, moderately, and guilt-free. Oh, and of course, to make exercise a part of your live forever.

FAT-STORING HABITS	FAT-RELEASING HABITS
dieting	giving up dieting
restricting fat and sugar	eating a variety of different foods regardless of fat and sugar content when you are hungry
skipping meals	eating five or six small meals a day

overeating when you do eat	eating moderately
eating the majority of your food intake at night	eating the majority of your food intake during the day
avoiding exercise	incorporating exercise

Don't diet, eat! Don't eat less, move more! Don't eat less frequently, eat more often! And your fat cells will become smaller over time with The Meno-Positive Approach to a Trimmer Transition.

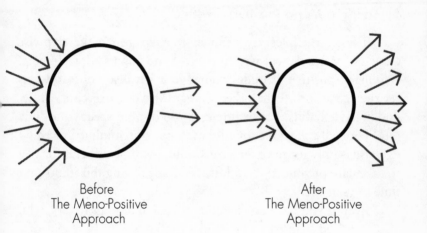

Before
The Meno-Positive
Approach

After
The Meno-Positive
Approach

I am usually philosophically against before and after photos—diets use them to lure you with the message "You, too, can lose fifty pounds and have a complete transformation like the woman in these pictures if you make out a check today for $119.95 (or three easy installments of $39.95)." What they don't tell you is that the woman was told to find the worst "before" shot she could, and prior to the "after" shot, she had a complete body makeover with a new hair style, makeup, and a crash course on accessorizing.

But, with the before and after photos of fat cells, it's impossible to "doctor up" the pictures. Fat cells can't be made up or camouflaged to look smaller or larger. Real, measurable changes occur. Whether your fat cells get 5 percent smaller or 50 percent smaller, they *will* shrink when you follow the five principles of The Meno-Positive Approach:

1. **Acquiring Meno-Positive Attitudes**
2. **Mastering Meno-Positive Fitness**
3. **Embracing Meno-Positive Eating Habits**
4. **Maximizing Meno-Positive Food Choices**
5. **Living a Meno-Positive Lifestyle**

These principles are ordered to help you make stepwise changes for permanent weight control and enhanced well-being. Acquiring positive attitudes comes first because your attitudes set the scene for all the other changes in your exercise, eating, and lifestyle habits. For example, if you don't respect your body (and yourself), view menopause as a loss of femininity, or think exercise is only for mice on a treadmill, it will be difficult for you to take care of your food and fitness needs during this important time in your life.

Even if you have an exercise attitude like Joan Rivers, who said, "If God wanted us to bend over, he would have put diamonds on the floor," I'll help you find your dangling carrot (or carat) to motivate you to move.

If you already have a positive exercise attitude and have been exercising for quite some time, your program may have reached its expiration date. It's no longer working, so you'll have to make some adjustments for it to work for menopause. You may have to exercise longer, add a different activity, or add some strength training.

Whether you're just starting an exercise program or are an exercise veteran, strength training will be a vital component because it's the only way to prevent the half pound of muscle loss a year. And by preventing muscle loss, you'll automatically prevent fat gain. The more muscle mass you have, the more calories will go to the muscle cells to be burned and the less will go to the fat cells to be stored. This is why incorporating exercise is primary and changing eating habits is secondary—but a close second.

When you eat, how often you eat, and how much you eat at any given time can also affect how much fat you store. Because menopausal women are highly efficient fat storers, it's imperative that we modify our eating behavior to match our new midlife metabolism. Your metabolism decreases during the transition, so your caloric needs decrease as well. This does not mean that you have to choose lower-calorie foods; it means that you have to choose *less* of *any* food. The amount you eat and the conditions under which you eat are more important than what you eat—even when it comes to fat.

For general health, it's a good idea to keep fat intake at a moderate level, but for managing menopausal weight gain, less fat in the diet does not necessarily lead to less fat in the fat cells. One study found that dietary fat accounted for only 2 percent of the weight gained by women in their mid 40s. The remaining 98 percent of the weight gained was caused by underexercising, overeating, and overactive menopausal fat cells.

If you are familiar with or are following the OFF Plan strategies in my first book, *Outsmarting the Female Fat Cell*, you are a step ahead. You will notice some similarities with The Meno-Positive Approach because you are already working with your female physiology and focusing on making your fat cells smaller. Now that you're in the transition, the OFF Plan simply needs to be fine-tuned to work for menopause—and you'll be well on your way to success.

THE SEVEN HABITS OF HIGHLY SUCCESSFUL MENOPAUSAL WOMEN

After working with women for over sixteen years, I have identified the following habits that are most likely to pave the way to success in managing weight, keeping excess weight gain at bay, and maintaining an active metabolism. The most successful menopausal women:

1. **Lost weight by themselves and for themselves.** They didn't do it at a weight loss center, and they didn't do it to please their significant other or placate their mothers. They did it to please themselves.

2. **Possessed a general acceptance of their bodies.** They didn't wake up each day hating their bodies, and they didn't spend hours every day feeling self-conscious about their bodies. Regardless of what they weighed, they felt good about themselves.

3. **Exercised regularly.** They were busy women, too, with busy schedules, but they found the time to exercise because it was important to them. To ease any athletic anxiety you may be experiencing, "regularly" did not mean exercising every day—four times a week was the average.

4. **Drank water throughout the day.** They didn't have just one glass at lunch or only a couple of sips when they walked by the water fountain. They always had water at their desk or carried a water bottle with them throughout the day.

5. **Ate regularly.** They didn't skip meals, forbid snacking, or eat the recommended three meals a day. They ate five to six small meals a day.

6. **Ate their biggest meal at lunch.** They didn't have a "liquid" lunch of Slimfast or carry around their own nonfat salad dressing for the noontime salad ritual. They ate real food: Chinese moo shu pork, spinach tortellini, chicken cordon bleu, meat loaf and mashed potatoes, or anything else they wanted.

7. Regularly enjoyed their favorite foods. They didn't give up mocha almond fudge ice cream, brie cheese, or fresh French bread with butter. They ate their favorite foods, they just didn't overeat them.

The bottom line is: *These successful women ate!* Think of someone you know who has maintained a naturally lean body. Your assumption may be that she's genetically blessed with a fast metabolism or that she carefully controls her eating by not eating. But, in reality, all or most of your leaner friends follow these seven habits without even thinking about it.

In addition to my clients or women you know, other successful women eat too! A recent study on the eating habits of 35- to 59-year-old women found that those who were most likely to maintain their weight during the midlife years ate four or more times a day and were *not* fat phobic—37 percent of their calories came from fat. That's even more than the national average of 34 percent of our calories from fat. Eating fat does not lead to weight gain, unless you overeat it.

You may think these seven successful habits are no scientific breakthrough, but I think they're one of the most significant finds of the century. I wish the six o'clock evening news or *60 Minutes* would report them so that everyone would discover the real nondieting, pro-eating way to manage menopausal weight successfully.

But what exactly determines success? It's not what the scale says or how much weight you've lost. Success is relative. Maintaining weight is success for some midlife women; slowing down weight gain is success for others; losing weight is success for those who were carrying too much to begin with.

My clients usually want specific numbers to grasp on to, so here's what I can offer. Of the hundreds of women I have tracked, they've gained an average of 2.7 pounds of muscle and kept midlife weight gain to about 5 pounds. Remember the average is 12 pounds, so they stopped weight gain in its tracks and cut the average by more than half. Many also lost a significant amount of weight; the amount being dependent on how much excess weight they gained to begin with. And they all reported more energy, improved body image, less food preoccupation, and no temptation to diet.

In my opinion, one of the biggest indicators of success is removing the word *diet* from your vocabulary and your life. I have been leading groups with a renowned therapist, Dr. Dee Tivenan, for many years now, and we've witnessed this transformation to diet-free living. When women say to us that "dieting would never cross my mind now" or "I'm truly listening to my body every day; that diet voice is gone forever," we know that they have achieved a healthier relationship between food and their bodies.

REPEAT AFTER ME: I AM NOT ON A DIET

To warn you ahead of time, I will be reiterating the need to stop dieting (and start exercising) throughout this book. Even though I briefly discussed the negative effects of dieting in the introduction and gave a more in-depth analysis on what dieting does to your midlife fat cells in chapter 2, I fear two important points may not have fully sunk in:

1. **Dieting causes megamenopause.** It intensifies and lengthens the transition.
2. **Dieting causes more midlife weight gain.** It increases the level of fat-storage enzymes.

We read all about the negative effects of dieting, the infinitesimal success rate of weight-loss programs, and the new antidieting movement. But we skim these articles to get to the "Get Slim for Summer" feature on the next page. Thousands of women have shared with me that they know they are not supposed to diet, but they are still secretively doing it. It has become so much a part of their self-identity that they can't (or don't want to) break free from the negative thoughts and restricting behaviors.

All indicators show that we are dieting more than ever before:

- The $30 billion diet industry has become the $33 billion diet industry in the past three years.

- On any given day, 30 million American women are on a diet. Are you one of them?

- We're still putting diet books on the best-seller lists and keeping them there for months and even years. We made the *Dr. Atkins Diet Revolution* a best-seller in the mid-1970s, and twenty years later, we put *The New Dr. Atkins Diet Revolution* on top again. Nothing much is new about it, including the inability to keep off the weight. Dozens of great nutrition books have been written that really do work, but unfortunately, they haven't gotten the recognition they deserve (a listing of these nondieting gems is included in the Suggested Reading).

- We're flocking to the diet doctors as never before. Last year, over 20 million prescriptions were written for diet pills. Any doctor can now be a diet doctor, and many are taking advantage of the lucrative opportunity.

If you are one of the millions still dieting, I want to make sure that you don't approach The Meno-Positive Approach as you would a diet. When I inform you that eating less at night will help shrink your fat cells, I don't want you to eat nothing at night thinking that you'll shrink them faster. Or when I tell you that exercising four times a week will produce the most fat burning, I don't want you to exercise seven days a week in hopes that you'll burn even more. That's what Elaine did. She took almost everything I said and turned it into a restrictive, destructive diet.

WHEN I SAID:	**SHE HEARD:**
Eat less at night.	Eat nothing at night.
Eat smaller meals.	Eat tiny meals (even a carrot stick can qualify)
Your caloric needs will eventually decrease by 400 calories a day.	I should count calories and eat as few as possible.
Exercise four to five times a week.	I should exercise as often as I can for as long as I can.
Give up dieting.	I can still diet as long as I exercise.

Like Elaine, many women think that they can cut calories and prevent the negative effects of muscle loss, lower metabolism, and regained weight—if they exercise. Even something as positive as exercise can't counteract the negative effects of dieting.

Researchers at Baylor College School of Medicine found that those who dieted and exercised regained all the weight they lost within two years. But those who exercised *without* dieting, maintained *all* their weight loss. **Dieting is the losing ticket any way you look at it.**

Dieting includes not only the traditional low-calorie plans and weight-loss programs, but also diet pills, fat-burning supplements, and the recent protein panacea. Let's discuss diet pills first. Redux and Fenfluramine (one half of the Fen-Phen combination) were recently taken off the market, so you couldn't take them even if you wanted to. And who would want to? The weight loss was not permanent, and the health risks were particularly alarming. They had been linked to sleep disturbances, nervousness, depression, abnormal heart valve functioning, and a potentially fatal lung disorder called pulmonary hypertension. Diet pills have never been the magical solution to weight loss. Any new ones that pop up in the future won't be the answer either.

Then there's over-the-counter chromium picolinate, the alleged fat-burning supplement. Celebrities have been spotted buying it. Politicians have been rumored to take it. Does it work? Does it really burn fat and build muscle? No, it doesn't. The University of Maryland has proven that exercise, not chromium, leads to muscle gain and fat loss. Those who exercised and took the chromium picolinate lost no more fat and gained no more muscle than those who just plain old exercised. Exercise always comes out the winner. **Don't waste your money on pills—invest your time in exercise.**

Eating protein is another recent dieting craze, but didn't we already do that in the 1970s? It didn't work then and it doesn't work now, but for some reason we think protein is the latest weight-loss breakthrough. There is everything from *The Zone* to *Protein Power* to *Doctor Atkins' New Diet Revolution* to a variety of others. In many of these plans, a baked potato can put you over the top. The culprit, they say, is insulin. One calls insulin a "monster hormone"; another calls it "the hormone that makes you fat."

The theory is that we are all insulin resistant, meaning that when you eat carbohydrates, excess insulin will be secreted from your pancreas, and excess fat will be stored in your fat cells (insulin is involved in the storage of fat). But what these books don't tell you is that only a small percentage of the population is insulin resistant, and for the rest of us, an oversecretion of insulin only happens when you *overeat* carbohydrates, not every time you eat them.

Some of my clients feel that they have given carbohydrates a fair shake and the bagels, pasta, and baked potato have let them down. So why not try the new high-protein diets? Because most of them are just diets. If you do lose weight, it's because the calorie and carbohydrate content are so low that your body is forced into ketosis, a massive effort by your body to make glucose from fat to fuel your brain and other organs. This is an unnatural and unhealthy state, and any weight you lose won't be lost for long. You'll gain it back—plus some.

On the positive side, these high-protein diets have sent the message that protein is an important nutrient. And as you'll learn in chapter 7, midlife women do need slightly more protein. But you don't have to go back to the diet plate of a bunless hamburger patty and a side of cottage cheese. You can have the bun and a side of satisfying fries because both carbos and protein are your pals—and *any* diet is your enemy.

THIS IS DIETING:	THIS IS THE MENO-POSITIVE APPROACH:
taking a pill	taking a natural, physiological approach
following a meal plan	following your body's eating plan
eating less than 1,200 calories a day	eating different levels of calories every day depending on how hungry you are.
eliminating or greatly reducing major food groups	eating a variety of foods from all the food groups
eliminating your favorite foods	incorporating your favorite foods

So repeat after me: *I am not on a diet*. Diets are unhealthy, unnatural, and unsuccessful for all women—but especially for midlife women. You are definitely not about to embark on a diet. Instead, you are about to begin a healthy, realistic, natural program to outsmart your menopausal fat cells. Are you ready?

THROW AWAY YOUR SCALE, BUT NOT YOUR COMMON SENSE

First things first: go into your bathroom, pick up that scale, and remove it from your life. As long as you are getting on the scale, you'll be functioning in the diet mode. You'll get down on yourself for gaining weight, restrict your eating to lose weight, and be discouraged when exercise causes a gain of muscle mass and overall weight. Pound for pound, muscle is one-seventh the size of fat. Gaining muscle doesn't make you a bigger person, gaining fat does.

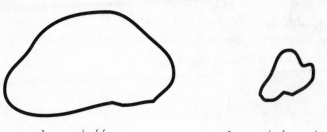

1 pound of fat   1 pound of muscle

I've had clients who stopped exercising because the scale didn't budge. But on closer analysis, they had lost fat, replaced it with muscle, lost inches, and often dropped a full clothing size. This is why I strongly recommend that you have your body fat analyzed before starting this program. A baseline measurement allows you to track changes in fat lost and muscle gained over time. Your health club, local YWCA, or yellow pages will direct you to where you can have it done. When you experience a gain in muscle mass, don't stop exercising—***stop getting on the scale***.

And use your common sense. Unfortunately, when it comes to weight loss, common sense is so rare that it should be called *uncommon sense*. Listen to your instincts: you know that diets don't work, exercise does, and the slower you lose fat, the more likely it will be a permanent loss. Your instincts will also tell you that *feeling good* is more important than *looking good*.

Studies have found that those women who start exercising or change their eating habits to look good don't last very long—six months at the most. But those who change their lifestyle to feel good, maintain their changes forever. **How you feel on the inside is more important than how you look on the outside.**

Looking good is an external motivator that is dependent on external validation—the compliments you get (or don't get) and the attention you receive (or don't receive). Feeling good is an internal motivator where the energy, mobility, and vitality you feel makes you want to keep feeling this way. Why do you want to lose weight? To look good or to feel good? For bathing suit season or for every season? To have more dating prospects or more mobility? To get thin or to get fit?

Why Do You Want to Lose Weight?

	YES	NO
1. To have the perfect body		
2. To please my significant other		
3. To be more successful		
4. To be happier		
5. To be more popular and well liked		
6. To be fit and healthy		
7. To move more freely		
8. To feel more comfortable in my clothes		
9. To reduce the stress on my joints and back		
10. To have more energy		

If you checked "yes" to reasons 1 through 5, then your desire to lose weight comes from external sources, and losing weight will not necessarily make you happier, prettier, or more popular.

If you checked "yes" to reasons 6 through 10, then your desire to lose weight comes from internal sources—and losing weight *will* make you more mobile, fit, and energetic.

What if you checked "yes" to all ten reasons? Then you want to look better *and* feel better. Don't worry, you have the internal motivators to balance the external ones, and being overly driven by looking good will diminish over time. Wanting to look good isn't unhealthy; being overly concerned with it is.

Even if you are more internally driven to get fit and lose weight, you still need to make sure that your goals are realistic and the way you go about losing weight is right for you. How can you tell if your goals are realistic? They are most realistic when they are not coming from the numbers on the scale, but instead by body fat analysis and how your clothes fit. Dropping a clothing size or a few percentage points of body fat is attainable for most midlife women, but fitting into a pair of size six jeans or reducing body fat below 30 percent is not.

If you are dead set on using pounds to set goals, they will *not* be realistic if:

- you want to weigh what you did when you were 20 years old
- you want to weigh what you did before you had children
- you want to weigh what you did when you were at your rock bottom weight (which was when you were on a 500-calorie diet)
- you want to weigh what the height/weight charts say you should weigh. (These charts may be accurate for some of you, but they don't take into consideration menopausal weight gain and the need to carry extra weight as we grow older.)
- you want to be at your "dream" weight—that magical weight where you will be swept away by your knight in shining armor

What is your "dream" weight? For Natalie, it was 125 pounds. A weight she hasn't seen since her high school prom.

What is your "happy" weight? Natalie answered that she would be happy with 135 pounds. A weight she struggled to maintain before her first child.

What is your "highest acceptable" weight? Natalie thought

for a moment and reluctantly answered, "I guess one-forty-five would be the absolute highest weight that I could bring myself to wear shorts in public."

I'm sure you know where I'm headed with this. If you must weigh yourself, forget about your dream weight, disregard your happy weight, and settle for your highest acceptable weight. The University of Pennsylvania studied sixty women who had lost a commendable thirty-five pounds, but none of them felt successful because they didn't reach their preconceived dream weights. Why do you think it's called "dream" weight? The only chance of achieving it is in our dreams.

So let's wake up, come back to reality, set realistic weight goals, and feel good when we achieve them. Throughout the five principles of The Meno-Positive Approach, the changes you make in your eating and exercise habits must be realistic as well. Continually ask yourself three important questions:

1. Does it make sense?
2. Does it feel right?
3. Does it feel good?

If it makes sense, feels right, and feels good—then it's a realistic lifestyle change. You are not expected to do everything recommended, but at the end of each principle, I'll ask that you choose which strategies you'll implement into your life. Use these three questions to direct your choices, and make one small change at a time.

The emphasis is on small steps. This bridge analogy may be helpful: Picture yourself at one side of a long bridge. Your ultimate goal is to get to the other side. At first, it seems overwhelming, far away, and out of your reach. You can't reach the other side in one big jump. You can't fly across the river, so your only alternative is to take one small step at a time. (If you have a fear of bridges, this analogy may not work very well. Picture yourself at the end of a football field instead.)

The first step is always the most difficult. But you don't have to worry about the first step because you've already taken it. You bought this book or borrowed it from the library or a friend. Each exercise session is a small step and each meal another, bringing you closer to your realistic goals.

It doesn't matter how long it takes you to reach your goals. That's why this is not a six-week program or even a six-month program. There is no endpoint. The Meno-Positive Approach is a lifetime plan, and it quickly stops being a plan and becomes the way you live.

What women want most during the midlife transition is to lose weight, discover more natural approaches to menopause, and find a good doctor. Good doctors are out there; start asking everyone you know. For the first and second desires, this is the most natural *and* successful approach to weight loss you'll find.

A TALE OF TWO MENOPAUSAL WOMEN

To help you get a feel for what you'll get out of this program, I will share with you two different women's experiences with The Meno-Positive Approach. One lost a significant amount of fat because she was carrying too much to begin with. The other gained some weight during the transition, but significantly less than the national average. Most likely, you'll identify with one of these two women.

Meet Suzanne: She's 41, a mother of two grade-school children, an exercise advocate, a speed walker, a moderate eater, and a relatively lean woman. She had maintained her weight at 132 pounds until about a year ago when her weight jumped 6 pounds. Her fear was that she would continue to gain 6 pounds a year and by the time she reached 50, she would weigh 186 pounds. But her fear was put to rest when three more years passed and she didn't gain another ounce. By changing her exercise program and eating habits, her weight gain was stopped in its tracks. She benefited most from eating her largest meal at lunch and using a Stairmaster for her aerobic exercise instead of walking. She had been speed walking for ten years, and her fat cells needed a different activity to force them to start releasing fat again. Suzanne may gain a few more pounds as she nears the end of her transition, but she now knows what to do to prevent excess weight gain, and she's prepared to accept another pound or two as necessary.

Meet Kathy: She's 53, an exercise advocate for everyone but herself, and has gained twenty-eight pounds since she entered the transition. She started dieting thirty-five years ago and has been on every single diet known to woman (even some that I had never heard of). She thought nothing would work for her because everything was working against her: her dieting past, her sedentary lifestyle, and her genetic propensity to be overweight. She wondered if The Meno-Positive Approach was even worth the effort, but she gave it a try anyway. Her efforts paid off—she lost sixteen pounds of fat the first year and kept them off for the rest of her menopausal years. The lightness she felt went beyond the weight loss; she felt better about herself, had more energy, and had fewer hot flashes. Kathy made many changes in her lifestyle: she started walking five times a week with a friend, she divided her daily intake into five small meals a day, she gave herself permission to eat her favorite foods in those small meals, and she completely gave up dieting. Her friends now call her a "reformed dieter." They joke about how she's always preaching about the evils of dieting, and they say that they are waiting for the day she walks into a restaurant and asks for the "nondieting section."

Why not institute nondieting sections at eating establishments? While we're at it, let's convert weight-loss centers to body-acceptance centers and turn our insatiable appetite for diet books into an insatiable appetite for knowledge. *Let's all become reformed dieters and informed eaters.* For Suzanne, Kathy, and you, the place to start is with your attitudes.

chapter four

ACQUIRING MENO-POSITIVE ATTITUDES

W*ithout putting much* thought into it, or worrying about grammar or sentence structure, quickly complete this sentence:

Menopause is _____.

How you described menopause gives an accurate first assessment of your attitudes toward the transition, revealing that you have an acceptance of it, anger toward it, or a sense of humor about it.

Your attitudes about every aspect of your life determine your actions each day, from whether or not you floss your teeth or wear a seat belt or laugh over spilled milk. Similarly, your attitudes toward menopause determine how you take care of your body and how you journey through your midlife years. For example, if you think that menopause is akin to the Wicked Witch of the West, then you'll waste so much time running away from it that you won't take the time to nurture your body and bring it back into balance. But if you think menopause is more like the insightful dog, Toto, following you wherever you go and trying to get your attention to alert you to what's behind the curtain, you'll travel through menopause with more intuition and awareness.

Here are some of the ways my clients have defined menopause:

- Menopause is always having to say "I'm sorry"—for forgetting people's names, blowing up at my family, and keeping my husband up at night with my insomnia.
- Menopause is a warning to stay away; all women should be given a sign that says "Beware of the Menopausal Woman."
- Menopause is like the T Rex in *Jurassic Park*—everyone fears me, you can feel my vibrations from far away, and my scream is deafening.
- Menopause is a fact of life; menopause happens.
- Menopause is no day at the beach.
- Menopause is a bitch.

These definitions are quite different from those found in the medical literature, but we can certainly relate to them. If you were to look up menopause in a variety of different dictionaries, these are some of the definitions you would find:

- the cessation of menstruation
- a disorder of estrogen deficiency
- a critical period or turning point in a woman's life
- a passage from one stage or state to another
- the point just before a fruit is fully ripened

Which definition do you most identify with? The only one I don't agree with is "a disorder of estrogen deficiency," but my personal favorite is "the point just before a fruit is fully ripened." It accurately says that the best is yet to come.

This description may sound great on paper, but applying it

to your personal situation may be seemingly impossible. Instead of a ripened, juicy, luscious plum, you may be feeling more like a prune. Or as Clara said, "I'm not feeling like a ripening fruit; I'm feeling like a fruitcake—the kind that nobody likes." Even if, like Clara, you are having a difficult time with the transition, integrating "the best is yet to come" philosophy can help. Knowing that the discomfort will diminish and life will stabilize can help adjust your current attitudes.

Let's further explore your attitudes about menopause. How do you feel about the transition, the changes in your body, and the changes in your mind? What is your menopausal mind-set? Take this questionnaire to find out. Circle the number that best reflects your agreement or disagreement with the following statements:

	AGREE				DISAGREE
1. Menopause is a disease requiring treatment.	5	4	3	2	1
2. Menopause is a marker of lost youth.	5	4	3	2	1
3. Menopause is "all in our heads."	5	4	3	2	1
4. I dislike my changing body.	5	4	3	2	1
5. My menopausal body is betraying me.	5	4	3	2	1
6. Gaining weight is a sign of weakness.	5	4	3	2	1
7. The best way to control weight is through dieting.	5	4	3	2	1
8. I have to eat low-fat foods to lose weight.	5	4	3	2	1
9. I'd rather diet than exercise.	5	4	3	2	1
10. I don't have the time to take care of myself.	5	4	3	2	1

The more you agreed with these statements, the more you'll benefit from this chapter and the remaining ones. The more negative your current mind-set, the more you will come to view menopause and its associated changes as natural and necessary, and the less you'll view it as a bothersome affliction.

MENOPAUSE IS NOT A DISEASE TO BE TREATED; IT'S A TRANSITION TO BE EXPERIENCED

If menopause were truly a disease, it would be classified as the most widespread female illness in history because it is guaranteed to occur in every single woman in the world. When we stop to think about menopause, we realize that it is not a disease of any kind, but from the time we were young girls, we were exposed to negative attitudes about this important transition. We watched as some of our mothers took doctor prescribed tranquilizers in the 1950s. Or we remember them reading the 1960s best-seller, *Feminine Forever*, which explicitly stated that middle-aged women were diseased from a lack of estrogen. For our mothers' generation, menopause was often thought of as a sickness that was only discussed behind closed doors.

Then, as we approached midlife, physicians of our own generation described menopause as "an unnatural state" or "a hormone deficiency disorder with massive medical and social implications." And the popular press and media have joined in to remind us repeatedly of the "symptoms" of menopause and the devastating effects they can have on our lives.

You may have noticed that thus far, I have successfully avoided using the word "symptoms." It hasn't been easy. "Symptoms of menopause" is an accepted, widely used phrase in medical circles, books, and support groups. With a thesaurus by my side, I have used the words "signs," "changes," and "discomforts" because I strongly believe that menopause is not a disease with symptoms to be treated. Rather, it's a natural stage of female passage to be experienced with knowledge.

The common signs of menopause are numerous and may, at first glance, seem ominous. Circle all that you are experiencing:

hot flashes	irritability	backache
dizziness	depression	headaches
fatigue	anxiety	joint pain
forgetfulness	mood swings	weight gain
sleep difficulties	thinning hair	menstrual cycle changes
increased food cravings	confusion	heart palpitations
constipation	diarrhea	waist expansion
sore throat	bodily hair growth	breast pain
frequent urination	facial hair growth	nausea

Like some of my clients, you may have been tempted to make one big circle around the entire list. Or you may have scanned this list and said, "What else is new? I've been experiencing these things since birth!" Maybe not since birth, but possibly since puberty. These signs are identical to what we may have experienced in puberty, PMS, pregnancy, and the postpartum period—the other times in our lives when our bodies were adjusting to changing hormones.

Unfortunately, most of the time we hear and read about only the negative changes during PMS, pregnancy, and menopause, but we can add some positive transformations to this list:

increased sex drive	increased productivity
increased creativity	greater awareness of your body's needs
greater confidence	enhanced communication skills
increased energy	improved self-esteem

I must acknowledge Margaret Mead for coining the term "menopausal zest" and reminding us that some midlife women do feel better than they ever have in their lives. There is also another phenomenon called postpartum pinks (the clever opposite of postpartum blues) where women experience a boost in mood following delivery. And premenstrually, some women report calmness and serenity instead of anxiety and stress (I wish I were one of them, for just one month).

But even if you are not one of these zesty, pink, serene women, the changes you experience during the different stages of womanhood are not symptoms of disease states. They are signs that your body is in a state of flux from changing hormones, and they are normal and natural characteristics of female passage. Sometimes these changes cause discomfort; sometimes they cause disruption, but they always tell us that we need to become more connected to our needs and that we need to be active participants in our well-being: that we need to rest, be alone, be with friends to share our feelings, be quiet, or be verbal. Menopause is our wake-up call, except you can't roll over and hit the snooze button. You have to get moving.

When women first notice some of the indicators of menopause, they often jump to the wrong conclusions: that forgetfulness is a sign of Alzheimer's, thinning hair of oncoming baldness, or headaches of a brain tumor.

Every change can be physiologically explained as the result of changing hormones. Even the hair loss. If you are a mother, remember what happened after you delivered your child? You hair seemed to fall out in handfuls. During pregnancy, the high estrogen levels caused you to retain more hair, and after delivery, the drop in estrogen caused it to fall out. If you monitored the hair loss throughout your monthly menstrual cycle, you'd also find that you lose more hair right before you start your period, which is when estrogen levels drop the most. Now that you are in the transition to menopause with a gradual decline of estrogen and other hormones, some hair loss is expected.

Similar explanations exist for every change in our bodies and minds. And if we search hard enough, we can uncover a positive aspect for each change, a beneficial reason for why it happens. For example:

- Weight gain is a way for your body to produce estrogen, feel better, and live longer (you already know this).

- Hot flashes may be a way to kill bacteria, boost our metabolisms, and/or burn off excess stress. With this explanation, you may wish for more hot flashes!

- Forgetfulness may be a way of de-stressing your life, helping you to overlook the little things so that you have more free time and brain space to focus on what really matters.

- Fatigue may be a way to force you to take a nap in the afternoon (especially if you're not getting enough sleep at night) or at least slow down enough to rest your body.

- Mood changes may be a way to connect to your emotional needs and begin to reprioritize your life.

One client challenged me with these positive explanations. "I defy you to give me a beneficial explanation for facial hair growth, especially my new mustache." Well, hair traps impurities and prevents infections, and these functions may become more important as we grow older. She thought she had a better explanation, "I think it grows to distract attention away from the hair loss on our heads, giving us something else to focus on so we won't be as obsessed with our receding hairlines."

Regardless of what you are experiencing during the transition and how you explain it, you have to trust that your body is undergoing changes for important reasons. And keep in mind that these changes will eventually subside. The hair loss will stop, the weight gain will stabilize, and the fatigue will diminish. Menopause will end—and you'll begin the next stage in your life.

Perhaps we need a better word to describe this pivotal time in a woman's life. Menopause is a clinical term that lends itself to a treatment approach. We call menstruation our period, which has helped to demedicalize our monthly cycles. Using the word *period* makes sense; it marks the end of our menstrual cycle as naturally as a period marks the end of a sentence. So what should we call menopause?

This very same question came up in conversation with a group of friends, and we had a few good laughs trying to think of an appropriate punctuation mark to represent menopause. We thought of a comma to indicate a pause just as it does in a sentence, but then thought better of it because it was too similar to coma and would give comedians too much material. We also considered a colon, but that had us on the floor doubled over in laughter.

Given the lack of medical research on women's health, we thought that a question mark may be the most appropriate, but the exclamation point gave menopause the emphasis it deserves—except we couldn't imagine women saying they were scheduling "an examination for their exclamation."

At the end of this lively exchange of ideas, we finally concluded that any punctuation mark was far too limiting because menopause really opens a whole new chapter in a woman's life. The word *menopause* is here to stay and so are the weight gain and other changes that go along with it. We have no other choice but to accept it and take responsibility for our own attitudes and how we experience our transitional years.

THE PLACEBO VS. THE NOCEBO EFFECT

Whatever you choose to do to help your body during the transition, do it with knowledge, conviction, and passion. That's the way to win at least half the battle. The more you believe in something, the better results you'll have. In other words, take advantage of the *placebo effect*.

The *placebo effect* means expecting a pleasant outcome, and because you expect it and believe in it, that positive outcome will likely occur. The *nocebo effect* is the opposite: When you expect a negative outcome, you'll most likely set yourself up to have a negative experience. During menopause, we are told that we will experience depression, anxiety, forgetfulness, and sleeplessness. Therefore, many of us believe we will experience all of them, and our expectations may come true.

The history of medicine is marked with the placebo effect. For centuries, consuming lizard's blood, frog sperm, and spiders were used with some surprisingly positive results. One of the most convincing examples of the placebo effect was demonstrated in the early 1900s. Ipecac was given to women to stop their nausea and vomiting. As you know, ipecac induces vomiting almost immediately, but because these women were told that this medication would help them—and because they believed it would—the ipecac had a 70 percent cure rate!

More contemporary studies continue to prove the power of the placebo effect. When researchers gave sugar pills to people with mild depression and told them that it was the latest and the greatest antidepressant, two-thirds reported that they felt remarkably uplifted. Then when the researchers warned that they shouldn't take two pills because the drug was so powerful, the sugar pill had an even stronger placebo effect. The active ingredient wasn't Prozac or Valium. It was hope.

The power of the mind is amazing, and as the ipecac and sugar pill experiments show, the mind can sometimes override the body. During the transition to menopause, the placebo effect can be just as powerful.

A number of studies have proven that those women who have positive expectations going into menopause have the most positive experiences. And vice versa, those with the most negative expectations have the most negative experiences. The Massachusetts Women's Health Study found that of the 70 percent who thought they would be depressed during the transition, the majority were indeed more likely to report depression.

One woman asked, "Does this mean that menopause is all in our heads?" Not if "all in our heads" means that it's solely psychological. Menopause is real with identifiable biological changes, but in a sense what's "in our heads" will affect our bodies. It may be unrealistic to ask you to wake up every morning proclaiming "Thank God I'm menopausal!" But how about waking up and saying, "I am in an important stage of my life, and I have the power to influence it positively."

You do have the power. Focus your mind and your body will follow: Believe that you can have a favorable influence, tap into the placebo effect, view setbacks as temporary, define menopause as a natural and normal stage of female passage, and when you are negative—catch yourself. Even if you are a "the glass is half empty" kind of person, you can transform yourself into an "at least the glass isn't completely empty" personality. Do whatever you can to view things from the most positive perspective possible.

You may be wondering if the placebo effect also applies to weight gain. That if you truly believe you won't gain weight during midlife, you'll keep your svelte curves for years to come. I wish it were that simple, but you can't completely will away weight gain. The changes in our fat physiology are too important for our well-being and survival. Nonetheless, the power of our minds can affect the power of our fat-storing biologies.

For example, if you think you'll gain forty pounds during the transition, it may become a self-fulfilling prophecy. You may set yourself up to gain forty pounds by overeating, not moving your body, and then saying, "See, I knew I'd gain forty pounds." The more appropriate comment would be, "See, my attitudes and behaviors set me up to gain forty pounds."

Instead, if you believe that you can prevent excess weight gain, then you'll be motivated to make the changes in your eating and exercise habits to lead you to that outcome. You may become more consistent with exercise and/or more conscious of your eating. And you can switch your beliefs in midstream as Kim did. At first, she was convinced that she'd gain thirty plus pounds in her 40s because both her older sisters did. And, sure enough, she steadily put on twenty-eight pounds by her 48th year. Then, after learning what she could do to change the physiology of her fat cells, her attitudes started to change. She realized that neither of her sisters exercised and both of them ate their way through the evening hours of prime time TV. She started to believe that she could make her fat cells smaller, and after a year of exercising and eating moderately, she lost fourteen pounds of fat.

If you've quickly done the calculations, you've figured out that Kim still gained a net of fourteen pounds—so where's the cause for celebration? That's another important component of acquiring meno-positive attitudes. Do what you can to minimize midlife weight gain, then accept your new healthy body and appreciate all that it's doing for you today and what it will do for you in the future. While you're managing menopausal weight gain, you also have to manage your menopausal body image.

MANAGING YOUR MIDLIFE WEIGHT CRISIS

I hope you're managing your midlife weight crisis better already. Just knowing the facts about your menopausal fat cells can bring you out of the crisis mode. You know the weight gain is not your fault; you know a good part of it is out of your control. But even with this knowledge, society's relentless pressure to remain thin and youthful can cause you to dislike your body, and thus yourself.

Disliking your body may seem quite normal. All of your friends make negative comments about their bodies. Weight, dieting, and eating are the most popular topics of conversation. Listen

to a group of women talking and see how long it takes for someone to bring up her thigh anxiety or waist worries. You'll find that
the majority of women in perimenopause are in weight crisis.

Are you in weight crisis? Answer "yes" or "no" to the following five questions:

1. Are you very concerned about your appearance and weight?
2. Do your concerns preoccupy you for a total of an hour or more a
   day?
3. Have your feelings about your looks caused distress or torment?
4. Have these feelings significantly interfered with relationships, family,
   occupation, or education?
5. Are there things you avoid because of your weight (i.e. social en-
   gagements, clothes shopping, the beach)?

Almost every woman I know answers "yes" to many of
these questions. If you answered "yes" to all five, then you may
have the extreme of poor body image called Body Dysmorphic
Disorder. It's a crippling preoccupation with our bodies where
weight loss is our number one goal and weight gain is our number one fear. This preoccupation directs our actions, eating behaviors, and lives.

Psychology Today recently conducted a readers' survey, and
one question they asked was "Would you trade five years of your
life for a five-pound weight loss?" A disconcerting 15 percent said
yes! Has weight loss become more important than living? *Glamour* did a survey a number of years ago and found that the majority of the 30,000 women polled would choose weight loss over
success at work and love at home. Has finding the magical solution to weight loss become more important than finding love?

In our society, thinness is overvalued, and we are led to
believe that achieving it is the vehicle to happiness, love, and success. Our obsession with thinness is reflected in almost everything we do—the foods we cook, the magazines we buy, and the

company we keep. It's also reflected in what we don't do—pose for a picture, swim in a pool, or make love with the lights on. It's so ingrained in our psyches that even the way we go about trying to manage our preoccupation reflects our obsession with it.

Some women try to manage their weight crisis through liposuction. According to the American Society of Plastic and Reconstructive Surgeons, liposuction is the number one cosmetic surgery. We submit ourselves to anesthesia, a six-week recovery, and thousands of dollars to have an average of three pounds of fat suctioned out. You don't walk into the surgeon's office a size 12 and walk out a size 8. In fact, your clothes may not fit that much differently. Liposuction works best for genetic deposits of fat that won't budge no matter how fit you are, but midlife weight gain is not genetic, it's essential.

Other women try to manage their weight gain by becoming elite athletes—marathon runners, triathletes, or centurion bicyclists. This amount of exercise may have never crossed your mind, and you may be more likely to opt for liposuction over in-line skating, but more and more of us are subjecting our bodies to hours of grueling exercise to try to combat menopausal fat.

And, of course, many women try to manage their weight preoccupation through dieting, which only puts more focus on our weight and makes us more preoccupied.

The point I'm trying to make is that we think the way to get rid of our weight troubles is to get rid of the weight. This thinking is faulty on two levels:

1. Losing weight does *not* decrease our weight preoccupation or improve our body image. Ninety-four percent of all women dislike their bodies regardless of their weight, and thin women are just as weight obsessed as larger women.

2. Weight is not the underlying source of our troubles; society's thin ideal and the pressure for thinness have put us in crisis.

The average American woman is now 44 years old—and in every way far from the typical 17-year-old model that defines the ideal figure. The only way the ideal is bigger than we are is in height. She's 6 inches taller. But we're 25 pounds heavier, six inches wider in the hips, six inches thicker in the waist, and three inches larger in the breasts.

	TYPICAL 17-YEAR-OLD MODEL	AVERAGE 44-YEAR-OLD WOMAN
height	70½ inches	64½ inches
hips	34 inches	40 inches
waist	22½ inches	28½ inches
chest	34 inches	37 inches

As long as we keep comparing ourselves to this thin ideal, we'll be in weight crisis. When you were 20 years old, it was virtually impossible to match this ideal. Now that you're 40 or 50 years old, less than 0.2 percent can match it. With these odds, it's not even worth trying!

These unrealistic ideals were once reserved for the under-30 crowd. We were that under-30 crowd—unhappy with our bodies and ourselves because we couldn't stay below 120 pounds for more than two weeks. Now, we're continuing to apply these impossible standards to our midlife bodies, and our unhappiness has turned to hatred. Recent studies have found that our body image is declining as we hit our fourth and fifth decades; whereas earlier studies showed that women were less concerned with their appearance and bodies as they grew older. Instead of welcoming self-acceptance into our mature lives, we are experiencing more self-deprecation.

It doesn't have to be this way. Women young and old are not emotionally predisposed to hate their bodies. This is a learned behavior, and we can unlearn it. Despite society's pressure to be thin, we can keep our perspective, focus on self-acceptance, and initiate a more positive body image during our midlife years.

Acknowledge the Impossibilities, Accept the Realities

The next time you compare yourself to a thin model or an emaciated picture in a magazine, remind yourself that:

- If a famine were to hit tomorrow, you'll survive; she won't.
- You're built like a woman; she's built like a 12-year-old boy.
- You have love handles; she has protruding hip bones that could cause injury.
- Thirty years from now, she may be laid up in bed with a hip fracture while you're laying down new soil in your flower bed.
- Not all good things come in small packages.

In the confines of your home, you may have a greater acceptance of your body, but as soon as you walk out the door, you may temporarily forget your newfound knowledge and attitudes (after all, memory loss is a sign of menopause). The diet ads bombard you, thin magazine models beckon you at the checkout counter, and all of your friends are talking about weight loss. While you're reminding yourself that thin is not necessarily better, also bear in mind the biological realities of menopause.

1. **Gravity does exist.** Everything drops about one inch by age 50. The only way to prevent the effects of gravity would be to spend your menopausal years on the moon.

2. **Middle-aged spread is real.** And the spread occurs mostly in the midsection, making elastic waists more and more desirable.

3. **Some weight gain is inevitable.** It's in your female blueprint, ingrained in your X chromosomes.

4. Getting your 20-year-old body back is impossible.
Even the Wonder Bra won't help.

We have no other choice than to accept these realities and acknowledge that who we are is more important than what we weigh.

Develop a Broader Sense of Body Image

Although for too many women weight has become the primary measure of how we feel about ourselves and our perceptions of how others view us, many other overlooked qualities also define body image. Circle all of the following words that you feel best describe your body.

healthy	graceful	agile
strong	dependable	soft
flexible	poised	cuddly
coordinated	balanced	sensual
quick	muscular	fit
curvaceous	playful	mobile
commanding	capable	sexy

Where are the negative words to describe our bodies? I purposefully left them out of this list. If you have only positive words to choose from, the only option is to evaluate your body positively. Gretchen felt that I tricked her with this list, then realized its benefit. Her assignment was to look at herself in the mirror every day and compliment her body with the words she circled. She reported that starting each morning with "My body is healthy, strong, muscular, balanced, sexy, and dependable" made a significant difference in how she felt about herself.

I'd like you to do the same right now. Go to the mirror and

say the words you circled out loud. Even if you are one of the 17 percent who admit that they avoid mirrors at all costs, I encourage you to try this activity—and do everything you can to avoid negative comments. Then be aware of how differently you carry yourself throughout the day.

Walk the Walk

When a woman feels good about herself and her body, it shows. She stands tall, walks confidently, and moves assuredly. And when a woman feels negatively about her body, it shows too. She slouches her shoulders, walks tentatively, and moves self-consciously. Interestingly enough, what we weigh has little to do with how we carry ourselves. Thinner women can fade into the crowd unnoticed while larger women can knock you over with their stately presence.

If weight were not a preoccupation and you were to live tomorrow body-positive, how would you be different?

Here's how one of my clients answered this question: "I would wear whatever I wanted to, probably a sleeveless top and fitted skirt that I normally wouldn't be caught dead in. I would walk into the office with my head high, stand with my arms open instead of crossed, and really throw my weight around to get what I wanted."

Take a day (how about tomorrow?) and throw your weight around:

- Imagine that weight is a positive quality, a vehicle to get what you want and make your presence known.
- Be bold—wear a sleeveless top or shorts and choose bright, attention-getting colors.
- Take a belly-dancing class—larger hips are an asset.
- Command the space you take up—look at Aretha Franklin; her figure is larger than society's ideal, but she carries herself proudly

and her presence can't be missed. It's her confidence and the R-E-S-P-E-C-T she has for her body that makes heads turn.

- Let your body do the talking—when you feel in command of your body and the space around you, notice how you communicate differently with others and with yourself.

Talk the Talk

Whether you realize it or not, you talk to yourself about a hundred times a day. You have internal dialogues—or you may even talk out loud—when you look in the mirror, get dressed, get on the scale, or walk into a party. Unfortunately, our conversations with and about ourselves are usually negative. Some common self-deprecating comments include:

"I'm so fat."

"I keep gaining weight; I'm out of control and disgusted with myself."

"I'll never get this weight off."

"I can't go out looking like this."

"They are all talking about how much weight I've gained."

When these or other negative thoughts enter your mind, try this technique: Visualize a Stop sign to make you stop deprecating yourself, then follow through with a more positive (or at least neutral) analysis such as:

"I'm not fat; I'm menopausal."

"Yes, I'm gaining some weight, but I'm not out of control. I'm a forty-five-year-old woman whose body is in complete control."

"I will get some of this weight off because I've started my lifelong exercise program."

"I can go out looking like this. This is my body, the only one I've got."

"The world doesn't revolve around my weight losses and gains; they're probably talking about something of real importance."

Weight used to be a much less important issue; fat used to be a normal part of body composition. In past centuries, a woman's belly could almost never be too round. In this century, it can never be too flat. Fat has become a sign of unhealthiness, laziness, and weakness—and a woman's weight has become a moral, political, and ethical issue.

To help reverse the way you think about fat and weight, a new way of thinking has surfaced. It's being called the "new paradigm," but it's not really new at all. I prefer to call it the "forgotten paradigm" or "the way we were." You can also use some of these alternative phrases for your positive self-talk.

THE CURRENT WAY OF THINKING	THE NEW WAY OF THINKING
Fat is bad.	Fat is just another way of being.
Large people are lazy.	Large people are just as active (or inactive) as thinner people.
Weight can be controlled.	Weight gained by dieting and overeating can be controlled.
Fat is unhealthy.	Any weight can be unhealthy, and any weight can be healthy as long as you're fit.
Large people overeat.	No significant difference exists in what people eat at various weights.
The goal is weight loss.	The goal is optimal health and self-acceptance.
Dieting leads to weight loss.	Dieting is a starvation state that leads to weight gain.
Fat is unattractive.	Beauty is learned.

Speaking of beauty, another thing you can do is start telling your friends that you have *calliopygia*. Some people may think it's a rare, contagious disease. It's not rare and it's not a disease, but hopefully it will become contagious. It's a Latin word meaning that you have "beautiful buttocks." Thousands of years ago when this word first originated, the bigger the buttocks, the more beautiful the bottom. Share this at your next dinner party; calliopygia is guaranteed to get an amusing response.

DIET HUMOR: GAINING A WHOLE NEW PERSPECTIVE

A potential client called me up and said she needed help quick. She needed to drop ten pounds in ten days to fit into her favorite cocktail dress for an important party. She asked me "What do you suggest I do?" I replied, "Buy a new dress."

I tell this story often. First for humor and second to reveal that there are alternatives to our "dieting crazies." Oh, and by the way, she did buy a new dress and had a great time without driving herself crazy on a ludicrous diet.

One of the best ways to change our dieting attitude is to laugh at ourselves and the dieting industry. I polled women on their most humorous dieting experiences. Here are a few of their stories:

- I've done more than diet. I bought an ear clip that was supposed to reduce my appetite, special underwear that was supposed to massage away my cellulite, and special shoes that were supposed to stimulate weight-loss acupressure points as I walked. The only thing that got stimulated was my anger—I spent over $100 on the most uncomfortable shoes I've ever worn.

- I was in for my annual exam, and after I got weighed, my doctor told me that I needed to lose weight and asked me if I was on a diet. I responded, "Oh yes! In fact, I'm on two diets right now." With a confused look, he asked why, and I answered, "Because one diet never gives me enough food."

- My best friend gave me a coffee mug that read, "All I want out of life are world peace and thin thighs." On the other side it said, "Actually, I really don't care that much about world peace."

- I was on a fasting diet to fit into my wedding dress and was so weak and malnourished that I passed out at the altar. My husband had to perform mouth-to-mouth resuscitation, giving "You may now kiss the bride" a whole new meaning.

- I got pulled over for running a red light, and the police officer asked for my driver's license. The picture was so outdated and the weight so grossly underestimated that he didn't believe it was me. I tried to explain to him that all women lie about their weight on their licenses and that I did weigh 115 pounds once after my most successful diet. It took me 30 minutes to convince him that the woman in the picture and me were one and the same. As soon as I got home that afternoon, I called up the DMV saying that I needed a new license. No, I didn't lose it. No, I didn't have a name change. I had a weight change to report. I need to provide my honest weight—please add 45 pounds for dishonesty.

- I was on an "all you can eat" fruit diet. This diet warned that the high fiber content may produce loose stools, but the correct wording should have been "liquid stools." I was in a job interview when it hit. I had to run out of the room screaming "Where's the bathroom?!" I was so embarrassed that I snuck out the emergency exit and set off the alarm.

Many diets are not just humorous, they're embarrassing—and sometimes foolish. You learned in chapter 2 that dieting clouds our thinking. With each diet, our methods become more senseless and our logic becomes more muddled. Here are some of the silliest questions I've received:

- Will the calories in toothpaste drip down my throat and cause weight gain?

- Will boiling my food first extract calories?

- How many calories do I burn chewing?

- If I let the ice cream melt before I eat it, will it have fewer calories?

- Does water flush out fat?

- If I exercise *in* the sauna, will I burn more calories?

- If I eat lunch *on* the stationary bike, will I burn up the calories as I eat them?

Perhaps you have asked similar questions or bought crazy gadgets. What extremes have you gone to? What's your most humorous diet story? Share it with a friend, ask your friends to share theirs with you, and have a good laugh on the dieting industry. Laughter can change your whole perspective.

IN MENOPAUSE WE TRUST

You can initiate a change in attitude for your change in life. You can shift from a negative outlook to a positive one. You can transform yourself from feeling powerless to feeling powerful. Here's how:

- **Call a truce with your fat cells.** Wave a white flag and start negotiating on their terms.

- **Call a truce with food.** Erase the "eat healthy or die" messages and reprogram your feelings toward food.

- **Call a truce with menopause.** Trust your female biology and let your body guide you to optimal well-being. It will tell you what feels good and what doesn't. Hating yourself doesn't feel good; accepting yourself does. Depriving your body doesn't feel good; feeding it does.

Your body will help you find the right balance to feel your best, and this balance will be achieved through a middle-ground, nonjudgmental way of thinking. Our choices are not as limited as we think. Many women have a bipolar way of thinking and evaluating themselves that prevents them from being at peace with their bodies and themselves. They believe they are either:

thin	or	fat
healthy	or	unhealthy
perfect	or	imperfect
youthful	or	old
fit	or	unfit
disciplined	or	undisciplined

With The Meno-Positive Approach, there is no black or white way of thinking or right or wrong way of doing things. The "right" way is different for each of us, and your body already knows what's right for you and how to lead you there.

You have more healthy wisdom in your body than all the medical libraries in the world. Throughout the remaining chapters it's important that you listen to your body's messages and trust that your body will bring you to a peaceful balance. Body language is real. Your body is constantly sending you signals through goosebumps, a yawn, a blush, hunger, thirst, fatigue, or a full bladder. These messages become even more apparent during menopause as your body directs you toward wellness. Listen to them.

As Christiane Northrup, M.D., wrote in her book, *Women's Bodies, Women's Wisdom*, "Many women have been knocked unconscious by the conflicting demands of our culture." Well, bring on the smelling salts. Let's become fully aware, trust our bodies, take a positive approach, and live as well as we can for the rest of our lives.

HOW WILL YOU ACQUIRE MENO-POSITIVE ATTITUDES?

In this chapter and at the end of the remaining four principles, I will ask you to choose what you will do to implement The Meno-Positive Approach. A number of suggestions have been provided to help you feel more positive about menopause and your midlife body, but it's up to you to decide which suggestions best fit your personality and lifestyle. As you go though this decision-making process, continually ask yourself these three important questions:

1. Does it make sense?
2. Does it feel right?
3. Does it feel good?

Check all of the following that make sense, feel right, and feel good to you, commit to them over the next few months, and you'll be on your way to acquiring meno-positive attitudes.

❏ I will be aware of the positive changes that go along with menopause and the beneficial reasons for everything I am experiencing.

❏ I will become an active participant in my well-being.

❏ I will think of menopause as my wake-up call—a time to become more connected with my body's needs.

❏ I will take advantage of the placebo effect by believing that I do have the power to affect my transition and my weight positively.

❏ I will acknowledge the impossibilities of the thin ideal.

❏ I will accept the realities of menopausal weight gain—it's real, necessary, and inevitable.

❏ I will set realistic goals, take small steps, and measure success by how my clothes fit and how I feel.

❏ I will investigate having my body fat analyzed so that I can measure changes in fat lost and muscle gained over time.

❏ Each morning when I look in the mirror, I will describe my body with positive qualities that have nothing to do with weight.

❏ I will take a day and throw my weight around by commanding the space around me, and I will continue to do this every week.

- ❑ I will engage in positive self-talk and visualize a Stop sign when I have negative thoughts about my body.

- ❑ I will share my most humorous dieting experience with a friend and have a good laugh on the dieting industry.

- ❑ I will call a truce with my fat cells, with food, and with menopause.

- ❑ I will trust my body's wisdom and let my body guide me.

- ❑ I will take the next step of mastering meno-positive fitness by reading the next chapter.

chapter five

MASTERING
MENO-POSITIVE FITNESS

You *always meant* to do it. You feel guilty that you haven't done it. You used to do it when you were younger. You know a lot of people who do it. Or maybe you *do* do it, but it's not something you necessarily look forward to. You even had all intentions of doing it yesterday—but you had to work late, your child had the flu, you got stuck in traffic, something came up—and the day just escaped you.

Of course the "it" I'm talking about is exercise. Some people love it; others loathe it, but just about everyone knows that their well-being depends on it. Ninety-three percent of us believe that exercise is the single most important health habit to adopt, but only 20 percent have made it a lifelong habit. A prime example of how knowledge doesn't necessarily translate into action.

Now is the time to take action. You need to move during your midlife years more than you have ever needed to before. Your menopausal body is depending on you to exercise in order to:

- **Fight fatigue.** Fatigue is always in the top three of any list of menopausal concerns, and menopausal women who work out regularly report 25 percent more energy that those who are sedentary.

- **Recharge your metabolism.** Exercise can boost metabolism by 8 percent, and the appealing result is that you can eat almost the same number of calories a day at age 50 as you did at age 30.

- **Reduce mental sluggishness.** Fit 60-year-olds think and react more quickly than unfit 30-year-olds. They also score higher in word and math problems and generally have higher IQs.

- **Sleep soundly.** Stanford University discovered that a moderate exercise program helped women fall asleep faster and sleep longer.

- **Stabilize your moods.** Whether it's during the premenstrual time or the entire menopausal transition, exercise releases serotonin and the endorphins, the brain chemicals that positively affect your moods. Fit women report significantly less depression, anxiety, and mood swings.

- **Diminish food cravings.** Those women who exercise report 39 percent fewer fat cravings and 22 percent fewer sugar cravings. Fitness is so satisfying to your body that previously craved foods become less appetizing.

- **Reduce hot flashes.** By helping your body to metabolize epinephrine and other heat-producing hormones, exercise has been found to curtail hot flashes as much as 50 percent. The average sedentary menopausal woman reports fifteen hot flashes a day while the average fit menopausal woman reports only eight.

- **Achieve greater mobility, balance, and agility.** You may not be worried about getting around today, but 15 percent of us have a walking impairment by age 50. Exercise tones your muscles, loosens your joints, and keeps you moving with ease.

- **Strengthen your bones.** Exercise is your bone savior, preventing premature bone loss or reversing damage that's already been done. Tufts University researchers have proven that fit women maintain their bone density throughout midlife while sedentary women lose at least 1 percent each year.

- **Reduce your risk of breast cancer.** The University of Southern California School of Medicine found that those women who exercised three or more hours a week through their reproductive years reduced their risk of breast cancer by 30 percent. What if your reproductive years have come and gone? A recent study reported in the *New England Journal of Medicine* found that the protective effects of exercise may be even greater as we grow older. Postmenopausal women who exercised for at least four hours a week had a 37 percent lower risk of breast cancer.

- **Reduce your risk of heart disease.** A study on 73,000 women clearly demonstrated that as activity level went up, heart disease risk went down. Another study found that active women cut their risk of premature death from heart disease by 300 percent.

- **Stabilize your blood sugar.** Exercise helps your body to utilize insulin and glucose and, therefore, reduces your risk of adult onset diabetes. If you already have diabetes, an active lifestyle may even help you control blood sugar without medication.

- **Live a longer life.** Two hundred fifty thousand deaths a years are attributed to a sedentary lifestyle. A study of over 20,000 men and women at The Cooper Institute for Aerobics Research in Dallas found that exercise reduced the risk of death from *all* diseases by an average of 50 percent. Another impressive study tracked 40,000 postmenopausal women and found that even as little as one hour of exercise a week reduced the risk of death by 24 percent.

Live longer, live healthier, sleep better, think better, feel better—*any way you look at it, exercise is the antidote for what ails you.*

What about exercise being the antidote for stubborn

midlife fat cells? Where's the evidence for exercise and weight loss? The evidence is so extensive and persuasive that it deserves more than a bullet.

If you want to do everything you possibly can to deter menopausal weight gain and combat midlife fat—EXERCISE! It's the only way to boost metabolism, stimulate the fat-releasing enzymes, and shrink your fat cells without compromising their ability to produce estrogen and enhance your well-being. Researchers at the Washington University School of Medicine followed women from the beginning to the end of the transition and found that those who were fit throughout their midlife years were leaner, stronger, and healthier.

	SEDENTARY MENOPAUSAL WOMEN	FIT MENOPAUSAL WOMEN
Body fat	38%	25%
Fat weight	59 lbs	33 lbs
Muscle weight	92 lbs	96 lbs

Look at these differences! The fit menopausal women had body fat percentages thirteen points lower, carried twenty-six fewer pounds of fat, and accumulated four more pounds of muscle. Nothing else can match these results. No food plan, no pill, no secret formula—only fitness.

When you become fit, your fat cells automatically become smaller. Each of your 30 billion fat cells learns that there is another existence. They don't have to function solely as fat-storage receptacles—they can also manufacture fat-releasing enzymes and shrink in size.

But it takes the right combination of exercise to make your menopausal fat cells fit and encourage them to give up stored fat. Aerobic exercise will manufacture the fat-releasing enzymes that trigger the emptying of fat into your bloodstream, and strength training will speed up your metabolism and condition your muscles to burn up that released fat.

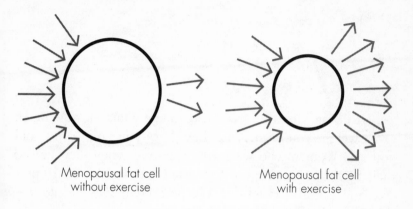

Menopausal fat cell
without exercise

Menopausal fat cell
with exercise

Exercise also encourages fat release in another way. It helps your body produce another source of estrogen so that your fat cells can willingly shrink without compromising your health. A recent discovery is that exercise stimulates your muscle cells to manufacture 25 percent of the estrogen your menopausal body needs. The more fit your muscles are, the more estrogen they'll produce, the less work your fat cells have to do, and the more cooperative they'll become in releasing fat. It's a win-win situation!

When you master meno-positive fitness by changing both your fat and muscle physiology, all variables work in favor of weight loss: a faster metabolism, more fat-releasing enzymes, more muscle mass, another source of estrogen production, and more cooperative fat cells.

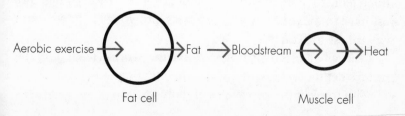

Aerobic exercise →   →Fat →Bloodstream   →Heat

Fat cell   Muscle cell

Has exercise anxiety set in yet? This is usually when my clients realize that a commitment to exercise is inevitable, and the "buts" start surfacing.

"But I'm too out of shape to exercise."

"But I'm too overweight to exercise."

"But I don't have time to exercise."

"But I'm too old to exercise."

It doesn't matter how out of shape you feel, how much extra weight you're carrying, how busy you are, or how old you are. Women who were 100 years old when they started their first exercise program increased muscle mass by 10 percent and overall strength by 170 percent. *If they can do it—we can too!*

STARTING WITH A CLEAN EXERCISE SLATE

Release any guilt you may feel for not having exercised, remove the word *but* from your vocabulary, forget everything you've ever heard about how you should be exercising—because this time it's going to be different.

During the fitness boom of the last decade, exercise meant work, sweat, and pain. We were either *Sweating to the Oldies* with Richard Simmons or sweating at the club with thin aerobics instructors in skimpy leotards. Now we're entering a new century, and you don't have to buy the latest fitness fashion, wear a thong leotard, join an expensive club, or sweat to anything. You just have to move and welcome fitness into your life in whatever way is best for you.

But what exactly is fitness? I like the World Health Organization's definition best: "Fitness is maintaining or developing the capacity to meet the challenges of daily life."

Those challenges may be physical, mental, emotional, or spiritual—and for menopausal women, all can occur simultaneously. Some days just getting out of bed is a challenge; other days accomplishing everything on our to-do lists before going to bed is our ambition.

I know what you're saying right now: "My to-do list can't handle one more thing to do. I barely have enough time to shower every day, so how can I possibly find the time to exercise?"

Time. It's the biggest reason we don't exercise. Fifty-seven percent of us say that we don't have enough time to exercise because of our jobs and 39 percent because of our families. But 21 percent of us say that we really don't have any excuse not to exercise. We find the time to do other things, yet we choose not to find the time to exercise.

To our credit, society doesn't make it easy to exercise. We could set the alarm for 5:30 A.M., but we may have three children to get ready for school and ourselves to get ready for work by 7:00 A.M. We could go to the gym at lunch, but we barely get a full sixty minutes for our lunch "hour," not nearly enough time to exercise, shower, eat, and make it back for a one o'clock conference call. We could exercise after work, but we may have an hour commute home, kids to pick up, dinner to make, and homework to supervise. We could do it at 9:00 P.M.—but by that time, we're too exhausted to move from the couch. Time is a legitimate factor working against us, but we also use it as a convenient excuse.

I've heard it all when it comes to exercise excuses: my puppy chewed my sneakers; I'm allergic to sweat; I'm a gymnophobic with a paralyzing fear of exercise. At least, I thought I'd heard it all until I heard Tara's excuse. "It's not my fault I don't exercise. It's my state's fault." Tara lives in Portland, Maine (my hometown) and had read a report from the Centers for Disease Control on the states with the lowest and the highest numbers of regular exercisers. The lowest: West Virginia, Mississippi, Kentucky, Maine, and North Carolina. The highest: Oregon, New

Mexico, Wyoming, Vermont, and Connecticut. Going along with Tara's rationale, I suggested moving from one Portland to the other.

It's not your state's fault, your dog's fault, or anyone's fault. We have to take responsibility for our level of fitness and make it a priority. We have to find our *internal motivator:*

- **Your motivator may be health.** Did the long list of benefits at the beginning of this chapter make you want to jump out of your reading chair and head for the gym you've belonged to for six years without ever having gone past the reception area?

- **Your motivator may be weight loss.** There's a good chance that this is what will drive you to the health club. It's why you bought this book. You may not have known that exercise would be so strongly encouraged, but you're into it now and realize that exercise is the only way to mastermind those midlife fat cells.

- **Your motivator may be a more positive menopausal experience.** Instead of calling the fire department to cool down your hot flashes, calling a personal trainer is the more effective solution. Exercise counteracts virtually all of the menopausal discomforts. It's a workout for your brain as well as your body, helping to alleviate depression, mood swings, and stress.

- **Your motivator may be someone else's tragedy.** Maybe you've witnessed the devastating effects of a sedentary lifestyle firsthand: a bedridden grandparent, a parent who can only walk with a walker, or an aunt with a broken hip. And your strong desire to prevent these disabilities will urge you to get fit.

- **Your motivator may be someone else's triumph.** Perhaps you have a friend or relative who has made the leap to fitness and is your inspiration. For Joan, her older sister was her exercise enthusiast. "A couple of years ago, my sister was so out of shape that she used to call herself an exercise 'misfit,' but now she's so energetic and active that we call her 'Miss Fit.' My goal is to follow in my sister's footsteps by walking my way to fitness."

• **Your motivator may be youthfulness.** Beth didn't get excited about the benefits to her heart, bones, or menopausal mood swings, but as soon as I told her that exercise could turn back her biological clock by fifteen years and make her body younger, she said, "Eureka! You just hit the motivational bulls-eye."

We all have an internal motivator, something that clicks to get us going. It could be anything: health, longevity, tragedy, vanity, even romance. Erma Bombeck has been reported to have said, "The only reason I took up exercise was so I could hear heavy breathing again."

Heavy breathing doesn't have to come just from the weight room. Physically active women also experience enhanced sexual activity. It doesn't matter *what* gets you moving—all that matters is that you *move*.

As we grow older and wiser, our motivation to exercise is higher than ever before in our lives. Women ages 35 to 54 are taking up exercise in huge numbers; more than any other age group. But our ability to stick with a program is at an all-time low. Half of all menopausal women who commit to exercise stop within six months of starting. How can we keep that initial rush of enthusiasm going and make a lasting commitment?

Commitment comes from knowing yourself—the type of person you are and the type of program that's right for you. If you choose a program that doesn't fit your personality and lifestyle, you'll be lucky if you last six weeks never mind six months or six years. What kind of exercise do you prefer?

• Do you like routine or spontaneity?
• Do you like to exercise indoors or outdoors?
• Do you like to exercise at home or at a fitness facility?
• Do you like making your own exercise schedule or making a scheduled exercise class?

- Do you like company when you exercise or do you prefer solitude?
- Do you like to exercise to music or in silence?
- Do you like competitive exercise or contemplative exercise?
- Do you like to exercise in the morning, afternoon, or evening?

How you answered these questions determines what type of exercise program is right for your personality: hiking in the woods, training for a race, group classes, or sunrise sessions. If you like peace and quiet, aerobics classes with heart-pumping music probably won't be for you. If you are a competitive person, taking a leisurely walk probably won't appeal to you. If you think that riding a stationary bike is the most boring thing you've ever done in your life, you'll come up with a million excuses not to put your seat on the seat. If your muscles seem to take longer to wake up than you do, schedule exercise later in the day. Experiment and you'll know when you've reached the exercise jackpot.

A lasting commitment comes from discovering your fitness preferences and realizing that you do have the time to fit exercise into your life. How many hours a week do you spend watching TV? The average person spends over twenty hours, so you could borrow a few hours from the sitcoms or exercise while you're watching a must-see show. How many lunch hours do you spend at a restaurant with a friend? Meet her at the park with a sandwich instead and go for a walk together. How much time do you spend reading the Sunday newspaper? Buy a reading stand for your stationary bike and pedal your way through the paper. No matter how busy your schedule, it's possible to find the time. Identify the ways you can "kill two birds with one stone," the days where you do have an hour to spare, and the time of day that you could work it in if you juggled a few things around.

Even though you may find the perfect time of the day for you to exercise and the ideal program for you, there's a good chance that someone will come along and tell you that you're going about it all wrong. Liz had been swimming for over a year when she ran into a self-proclaimed fitness expert who changed her whole exercise program. "I was loving my evening swims, but then I was told that swimming makes you fat and the only time to exercise is first thing in the morning. So I quit swimming and tried running at the crack of dawn. That lasted less than a week, and I haven't exercised since."

Everyone has their own opinion on how you should be exercising. Your partner may give you advice, your best friend may tell you what worked for her, and a magazine article may say something completely different. Only you'll know when your midlife body is thankful for fitness. Don't second-guess yourself—know yourself, trust yourself, and educate yourself on the myths of exercising. Here are the top ten fitness misconceptions:

1. **Exercising in the morning burns more calories.** Exercising any time of the day burns the same amount of calories. There is no "better" time to exercise.

2. **Swimming makes you fat.** When will we stop believing this one! Swimming burns fat as efficiently as any other aerobic exercise. If you need proof, check out the bodies of professional swimmers or hop in and give it a try. It's not as easy as you think to propel your body through water.

3. **The stair-climbing machines give you a big bottom.** About a year ago, this hit the news wire and women started bypassing the Stairmaster. It only lasted a day before it was refuted, but we still remember it. The stair-climbing machines give you a shapely buttocks, not a big one.

4. **Lifting weights will cause you to bulk up.** Bench-pressing 150 pounds may cause overdevelopment of muscles, but lifting lighter weights will not. Remember: muscle is dense tissue—one-seventh the size of fat. Strong muscles mean a smaller body.

5. **Sit-ups taper your waist.** A million sit-ups won't give you the nineteen-inch waist you may be striving for. Spot reducing has always been a myth, but that doesn't mean sit-ups are a waste of

time. By toning the muscles underneath the fat, you'll have a stronger back, better posture, and a slightly smaller waist because the muscles will become more compact.

6. **If you don't exercise, muscle turns into fat.** It's impossible for muscle to become fat, but it's very possible to lose muscle and gain fat in its place—which is exactly what happens when you're sedentary.

7. **Exercise curbs your appetite.** You may not be hungry right after your workout because endorphins reduce your appetite, but you may be hungrier later. Because exercise boosts your metabolism and caloric needs, you may experience an overall increase in appetite and daily food intake *while you're losing weight.* Fit menopausal women eat more *and* weigh less.

8. **Exercise produces an immediate burst of energy.** We are often told that the reward of exercise is enhanced energy and productivity right after, but many people don't feel it and start to lose their motivation. It's not necessarily how you feel immediately after; it's the increased energy and well-being you feel twenty-four hours a day.

9. **Men are better athletes than women.** Men start off with more muscle, larger hearts, and more blood volume, but with training, we can become just as fit as men. We are running marathons, climbing mountains, and competing in sports as never before.

10. **Walking is the best form of exercise.** As you'll discover, other forms of exercise are as good, if not better, for midlife women to release a significant amount of fat. Some perimenopausal women find that they are still gaining fat even though they are walking for hours every week.

Denise had been walking for thirty minutes every day for the past ten years. In our first session together, she voiced her frustration with weight gain despite her infallible commitment to exercise. And she voiced her surprise when I suggested that she take a break from walking for a while and find another form of exercise she enjoyed. Within a month of cycling on a bike path four days a week for an hour (because she loved the outdoors and couldn't imagine herself staring at a wall on a stationary bike), her body finally started to give up fat again.

TAKE A BREAK FROM WALKING

Walking can be a great form of exercise, but your menopausal fat cells are not going to let a thirty-minute walk around the park get the best of them. Our bodies are ergodynamically designed to walk. The way our muscles and tendons attach to our bones allow ease of movement with the "one step in front of the other" routine. It's automatic and relatively effortless. A little too effortless for some of us to lose fat.

If you're just starting an exercise program, walking will give you all the fat-burning benefits you are searching for. Since the Industrial Revolution and the invention of the automobile, escalator, and elevator, most likely you don't walk to work, walk to the store, or walk up the stairs very often. Your body isn't used to walking, and your fat cells will be sufficiently challenged to release fat. (Remember this section five or ten years down the road.)

If you've been walking as your form of exercise for the past ten or more years and are still gaining fat, I regret to inform you that you're probably due for a change. You have one of two choices: alter your walk or add a new activity.

Because walking is enjoyable to many women, here's what you can do to make walking work for menopause:

- **Change your route.** If you've been doing the same walking trail since it was installed in 1985, your body knows every turn, tree, rock, and house along the way. Find another trail and go somewhere completely different. Your fat cells will say, "Hey! I don't recognize this route. It may be harder or longer than I'm used to, so until I know, I better donate some fat for back-up energy."

- **Head for the hills.** Most women walk on relatively flat ground and at a relatively moderate pace. Walking uphill is harder; the steeper the incline, the harder your muscles, heart, lungs, and fat cells have to work to push your body up the hill. To protect your knees, try to avoid steep downhills and keep your knees bent to cushion the downward impact.

- **Search for stairs.** Walking up stairs uses different muscles from those used when walking on the ground. Find a building with a lot of stairs, or maybe a football stadium with many bleachers, and make it a part of your route—and part of your routine. Think Rocky Balboa and throw your arms up in victory when you reach the top.

- **Put some pep into your step.** Your arms determine your pace; keep them at a ninety-degree angle close to your body and move them faster to quicken your stride. At least three miles an hour is the pace it takes for walking to whittle away fat.

- **Develop a walk/jog routine.** Jogging is a whole different form of exercise from walking. You don't have to become a long distance runner (unless you want to), but breaking into an occasional jog while you're walking will break down some additional fat in your fat cells.

- **Become a pack walker.** When you first start walking, your muscles and bones are not used to carrying your body weight. At first it's difficult, but then your body gets used to moving your weight with each step. Adding an additional five or ten pounds with a backpack full of sand or newspapers can make you feel like you are walking for the first time again. If you have back problems, however, this technique is not advised.

Any of the above suggestions will help direct you down the walking path of fat loss. The other option is to take a break from walking and try a different activity. You can still walk a couple of times a week, but also add something that you've always wanted to do. The only prerequisite is that it also has to be aerobic, an activity that uses your major muscle groups in a rhythmical, nonstop fashion.

Take up swimming. The fitness boom has pretty much ignored swimming, but over the past few years the number of midlife women swimming has doubled. When I suggest water sports, many of my clients think back to childhood when they loved playing in the water. Some have turned to the water because it's easy on the joints and back. Others dive in for the soothing feeling of being in the water. Instead of swimming laps with the crawl or breast stroke, many women have found their niche in aqua aerobics.

Try rollerblading, step classes, cross-country skiing, jogging, cycling, using a piece of exercise equipment, or an exercise video. When I mentioned exercise videos to Anne, she rolled her eyes and said, "I've got over forty of them in my video library, and I've watched every one of them from the recliner in my family room. Many of the instructors are too perky, and many of the moves are too complicated. When their arms go up, mine go down. When they move left, I go right. I feel humiliated by a six-inch figure on the screen."

Exercise videos were obviously not for Anne. But if you haven't given them a try, rent a few and see what you think. When you're short on time, they can come in handy.

Each type of exercise you choose uses different muscle groups—increasing your ability to burn fat. When you do the same activity over and over again (whether it's walking or swimming or cycling), your muscles and fat cells get complacent. The movement becomes too easy for them, and they yawn when you change into your workout attire.

That's why patchwork exercise is best—mixing and matching different activities. This is also called cross-training, and it's in vogue right now for good reason. It speeds up fat burning, prevents boredom, reduces wear and tear on muscles, and leads to total body fitness. Runners cross-train by cycling.

Cyclists cross-train by rowing. Swimmers cross-train by running. Everyone can cross-train by doing more than one activity. *You* can cross-train by mixing and matching different forms of exercise: walk one day, swim another, cycle on another, and every now and then throw in some other activities. **The magic bullet for menopausal women is doing more than one activity.**

IT'S ALL IN THE TIMING

We've covered the "what" form of exercise to do, now for the "how": How often, how long, how hard? The American College of Sports Medicine recommends three to five times a week for twenty to sixty minutes at 60 to 90 percent of your maximum heart rate. That's a broad guideline. Let's narrow it down.

The men in your life will fare well with three times a week for twenty minutes at any intensity. Their fat cells respond so quickly to exercise that they release fat within minutes of movement. One of my more humorous clients calls the male response to exercise "premature fat cell ejaculation."

The female response to exercise takes significantly longer. As a premenopausal woman, three times a week for forty-five minutes most likely did the trick for you to release fat from your fat cells. But now that you are in the transition to menopause with extra-stubborn fat cells—four times a week for sixty minutes is probably what it will take for your fat cells to get stimulated.

This may sound like a lot of exercise, but our midlife fat cells are so stubborn that we have to coax them to release fat. For the first thirty minutes or so, your fat cells are ignoring you. Your muscles are using glucose as their primary energy source because it is is stored in your muscle and is right there ready to be burned. Fat is stored away from the muscle (next to the belly button or in the inside of your thighs), so it has to be first released and then travel to your muscle to be burned. Because our midlife fat cells take longer to release the fat, exercising the full sixty minutes will give them all the time they need to release fat and direct it to the muscle to be burned.

Patience, consistency, and perseverance are what it takes for midlife women to become efficient fat burners. If you're just starting, inform your physician of your exercise plan and get any tests he or she recommends. Then pace yourself and progressively add time to work your way up to sixty minutes. In the beginning, ten or fifteen minutes will prepare your body to release fat in the future, and smaller doses of exercise will still boost your metabolism.

Whatever exercise you choose and however long you do it, *never* get out of breath. The word *aerobic* simply means with oxygen. Every fat cell needs oxygen to release fat, and if you push yourself too hard and are huffing and puffing, you render your body incapable of burning fat because your fat cells are deprived of the necessary oxygen. Monitor your rate of breathing and keep the intensity moderate. You want your breathing to be increased, but not so much that you couldn't carry on a conversation. You can also monitor your heart rate to make sure you're in a moderate training zone—consult an exercise professional on how to take your heart rate and how many beats per minute defines your training zone.

Sixty minutes of aerobic activity four days a week at a moderate intensity—that's part one of mastering menopausal fitness. Now for part two.

HUSTLE TO BUILD MUSCLE

Over the last few years, exercise physiologists have come to a startling conclusion: aerobic exercise is great for the heart, lungs, and fat cells, but it doesn't stop the muscle loss that occurs with aging. Those who walk or cycle or row into their 70s lose almost as much muscle mass as those who are sedentary. We've been so consumed with aerobics that we've forgotten the other component of fitness—maybe the most important for your menopausal body—*strength training*.

Aerobic exercise is vital to stimulate fat loss during perimenopause—that's why I discussed it first. But you have 639 muscles in your body that also have to be stimulated. Which do you think is the strongest muscle in your body? No, it's not your thigh muscle or your buttocks or your biceps. The strongest muscle is the one you use most often, many times a day whether you're sitting, standing up, or even lying down. It's your jaw muscle, and it's three times as dense as any other muscle in your body because of all the chewing it has to do.

The goal is to work the other 638 muscles with as much dedication and consistency as you work your jaw muscle. By adequately working as many muscles as you can with strength training, you'll not only gain muscle mass and strength, you'll also lose more fat than with aerobics alone. Here's why:

- **You'll store less fat when you eat.** More of the calories you eat will go to your muscle mass to be burned instead of to your fat cells to be stored. Strong muscles burn 75 percent of your caloric intake morning, noon, and night.

- **You'll burn more fat when you exercise.** Once fat is released from your fat cells with aerobic exercise, fit muscles will more effectively ignite the fat and use it for energy.

If you choose not to integrate strength training into your exercise program, you'll continue to lose a half pound of muscle a year. But with strength training, this can be 100 percent prevented, and any muscle you've already lost can be 100 percent regained. There are no maybes or ifs or probablys—it's definite—and it's fast. Within three months, you'll notice about a 20 percent increase in strength. And within a year, you'll gain about three pounds of muscle and increase your strength by 76 percent!

Your bike rides or step classes or morning walks will increase muscle mass and strength to an extent, but you have two types of muscle fibers in your body: slow twitch and fast twitch. Slow twitch muscle fibers contract slowly and repetitively under little resistance. They give you endurance and stamina and are called upon for your aerobic exercise. Fast twitch muscle fibers contract quickly and explosively in response to heavier resistance such as lifting a heavy object, catching oneself in a fall, doing wind sprints, or swinging a tennis racket.

We've done a great job with the slow twitch muscle cells via aerobic exercise, and we've received the benefits in unclogging arteries and lowering blood pressure, but most of our fast twitch muscle fibers are out of shape despite our years of exercise. This is unfortunate because the fast twitch muscle fibers increase your metabolism even more than the slow twitch fibers. The most effective way to raise your metabolic rate and calorie-burning potential is to stimulate your fast twitch muscle fibers with strength training.

You don't necessarily have to join a gym and work the weight machines with one hundred other people to strength-train. The benefit of the machines is that they automatically get you into the right posture so that you don't have to worry about positioning. But you can also play tennis, racquetball, squash, bocce ball, basketball, or softball. Or you can golf, canoe, kayak, sail, bowl, do floor exercises, or take a karate class. All of these exercises involve either stop/start movement or lifting an object, and all of these exercises strengthen your muscles. You don't even have to leave your own backyard. Gardening is one of the best all-around strengthening exercises because it uses many different muscles with raking, bending, weeding, planting, bagging, and hauling. Neither your body nor your backyard will ever be the same.

In addition to the weight machines and strength building sports and hobbies, a popular option is weight lifting with hand and ankle weights, or, as they are often called, free weights. They're not free in cost (although they are inexpensive), but they do free you from cumbersome equipment. When some of my clients first get interested in free weights, they are confused by the lingo. I had a British client who thought a "lift" was an elevator (in England it is, but the only muscles you use are those in your index finger when you push the button), a "rep" was a salesperson for a product line, and a "set" was a victory playing cards. All true again, but here are some other definitions:

- A *lift* is simply lifting the hand or ankle weight—a complete move up and down.

- A *rep* is a series of lifts—the number of times you repeat the movement before you move on to the next lift.

- A *set* is the total number of repetitions of all the different lifts.

The recommendation is to do at least two sets of eight to twelve reps two days a week. If you hit the major areas—biceps, triceps, shoulders, chest, hips, buttocks, thighs, and calves—it will take about thirty minutes to complete two sets of these eight lifts.

SET 1

8 to 12 reps of the bicep lift

8 to 12 reps of the tricep lift

8 to 12 reps of the shoulder lift

8 to 12 reps of the chest lift   pause

8 to 12 reps of the hip lift

8 to 12 reps of the buttocks lift

8 to 12 reps of the thigh lift

8 to 12 reps of the calf lift

SET 2

8 to 12 reps of the bicep lift

8 to 12 reps of the tricep

8 to 12 reps of the shoulder lift

8 to 12 reps of the chest lift

8 to 12 reps of the hip lift

8 to 12 reps of the buttocks lift

8 to 12 reps of the thigh lift

8 to 12 reps of the calf lift

Unlike aerobics, these sets and the thirty minutes do not have to be done all at once. You can break up the different lifts and spend ten minutes in the morning, ten minutes at lunch, and ten minutes at night. Or you can do the upper body lifts today and the lower body lifts tomorrow. You need at least a day in between working the same muscle groups to repair the muscle and get stronger. If Saturday and Sunday are your only options for strength training, do it early Saturday and late Sunday to leave as much time as possible in between sessions.

The advantage of using free weights is that they are easy and convenient. You can use them while you're watching TV or talking on the phone. You can use them at home or at work. Here are some general guidelines:

- Get an okay from your doctor before you start strength training or any type of exercise program.

- Get the equipment you need: multiple pairs of dumbbells—three-, five-, eight-, and ten-pound hand weights and ankle weights that you can add up to twenty pounds.

- Everyone's starting weight is different depending on level of fitness. Find a weight that you can lift between eight and twelve times. If you start with five pounds but find you can lift it only five times, drop down to three pounds. If you start with five pounds and find you can lift it fifteen times, go up to eight pounds. Begin with the lowest possible weight, and as you become stronger, adjust the weight accordingly.

- Follow the 3-1-3 technique; lift slowly up for three seconds, pause for one second, and take three seconds to bring the weight down slowly.

- Breathe—exhale as you lift up, inhale as you go down.

- If you feel pain, stop. A slight burning sensation is normal and actually a sign that you're working your fast twitch muscles, but a sharp pain in your joints or muscles is a sign that you're doing the movement improperly or the movement is not right for your body. This is especially true if you have back or joint problems.

- Get expert guidance to get expert results. Visit a reputable gym for instruction, buy a good book that gives detailed guidance (Miriam Nelson's *Strong Women Stay Young* is excellent), or find a certified personal trainer who can tailor strength-training exercises to your body.

Personal trainers aren't just for celebrities anymore. Dozens of my clients have sought their expertise either to get them set up or to keep them motivated. Depending on where you live, the fee can range from $25 to $100 an hour. Think of it as an investment in your health or a birthday present for your body. Ask your friends for referrals or call the following organizations:

American Council On Exercise (ACE)	619-535-8227
Aerobics and Fitness Association of America (AFFA)	800-968-7236
International Association of Fitness Professionals (IDEA)	800-999-IDEA
The Fitness Connection	800-318-4024

To master menopausal fitness, you need both the aerobics and the strength training. Four hours of aerobic exercise a week will ensure fat release and one hour of strength training will guarantee muscle gain and a faster metabolism. You'll also increase overall strength by 76 percent, improve balance by 14 percent, and feel and look fifteen years younger. Tufts University is to be congratulated for this groundbreaking research. Their most publicized result was that after just one year of strength training, the bone density, muscle mass, and activity level of 60-year-old women were comparable to 45-year-old women. Because youth and activity go hand-in-hand, these women also became 27 percent more active in their daily activities without being instructed to do so. They took the stairs more often, walked around more, gardened more—even cleaned house with more vigor.

Activity leads to more activity, creating an upward spiral of fitness. By moving your body and gaining muscle, you become stronger, desire even more activity, do more activity, and become even stronger.

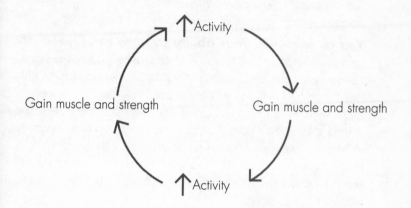

As one of my clients said, "This all makes complete sense to me. I'll just turn that upward spiral of activity into a training tornado. I'll cross-train every day, lift weights every day, do jumping jacks while I'm waiting for the bus, do pelvic tilts while I'm waiting at traffic lights, do sit-ups while I'm watching TV, and do leg lifts while I'm talking on the phone. By the time I'm done, I'll be active sixteen hours a day."

Be careful. More exercise is better—until it becomes too much for your body to handle.

EXERCISE SMARTER, NOT HARDER

There is no reason in the world to exercise more than four hours a week aerobically and one hour a week with strength training. Actually, there are many compelling reasons *not* to go overboard with exercise:

- **You increase your chances of injury.** An over-40 body is less resilient than a younger body. If you go too fast, push yourself too hard, or don't take days off to heal and recuperate, muscles can become overstimulated, and minor injuries can become chronic and debilitating. Some women bring the same compulsive behavior to exercise that they have with food and dieting. Binge exercise can be just as destructive as binge eating.

- **You compromise your ability to burn fat.** Overexercise (usually defined as ten hours or more a week) causes a starvation response similar to dieting. When your menopausal fat cells feel threatened with too much exercise, they hold on to their fat for survival. Adding more exercise does not necessarily speed up weight loss; it may have the opposite effect and slow it down. When my overexercised clients reorganize their program to a moderate level with four hours a week of aerobic and an hour of strength building, they are surprised to discover that they become leaner with less activity.

- **You compromise your immune system.** According to research from the USDA, too much exercise reduces immune function by 20 percent. When overexercise is combined with undereating, immunity drops by 50 percent, making us twice as susceptible to colds, flus, and infections. Studies done on long-distance runners have found that those who run more than sixty miles a week are twice as likely to get sick as those who run twenty miles a week.

- **You compromise your sleep patterns.** Exercise is a stimulant, and too much, especially later in the day, can cause increased wakefulness and fragmented sleep at night. Moderate exercise helps you fall asleep, but overexercise can prevent you from falling asleep.

- **You compromise your longevity.** The Cooper Institute in Dallas found that moderate exercise decreased death rates in men and women, but overexercise increased death rates for women only.

• **You compromise your skeletal system.** Calcium is used by the muscles for each contraction and is also lost in sweat. With extreme exercise, up to 3 percent of your bone mass can be lost in one year. But with moderate exercise, you can gain up to 1 percent a year.

As you can see, too much exercise can produce the same problems as too little. The point is that you can get too much of a good thing. Moderate exercise is what burns fat, boosts immune function, helps with sleep, and strengthens bones. And to get the full benefit of strong, dense bones, women have another consideration with exercise: To reduce your risk of osteoporosis, you also have to make sure at least some of what you are doing is weight-bearing exercise.

"Weight bearing" simply means carrying your weight over a distance, forcing your bones to become stronger as they carry that weight. When the first astronauts ventured into space, an unanticipated side effect was bone loss. Within a few days of total weightlessness, their bones became weaker and less dense.

Partial weightlessness occurs in the water. You weigh 75 percent less in the water than you do on land (weighing less may sound pretty good and you may fantasize about living in the fabled underwater city of Atlantis, but it's not so good for the bones). Have you noticed how easy it is to jump up or pick someone up when you are in the water? The water, not your bones, holds up your weight. Although swimming is still a great aerobic exercise, it's not considered a weight-bearing exercise.

Is walking weight bearing? Absolutely! Each step carries your full body weight forward. Is bike riding weight bearing? Not nearly as much as walking. With a stationary bike, you are sitting, so the bike seat is holding up your weight. If you mountain-bike up hills, it's a different story. Your weight shifts quite a bit and you often stand to propel the weight of your body and your bike up hills.

What about cross-country skiing? Outdoors and in the woods, yes. But with the indoor machines not as much as you might think. Your hips are stationary, resting up against the padded support structure, and your legs slide along the grooves. You are not really carrying your weight over a distance; you are sliding your feet in a stationary position.

Any activity that forces your bones to carry weight—your own body weight or the weight of an object—is weight bearing. The top five weight-bearing activities are gardening, weight lifting, house cleaning, dancing, and walking or jogging. This is why female movers, delivery people, contractors, gardeners, and house cleaners have some of the strongest bones in the world.

I've had a number of clients who have said, "I don't have to worry about weight-bearing exercise because I'm on hormone replacement therapy." HRT alone may not produce a significant increase in bone density, but HRT combined with weight-bearing exercise can increase bone mass up to 8 percent. Since women lose 1 percent of their bone mass each year from the mid-30s on, that reverses bone loss by 8 years!

Estrogen does work as a helper to deliver calcium to your bones, but your bones have to be in a position to accept it. Exercise places the right kind of stress on our bones to make them eagerly take in all the calcium they can get.

To achieve total midlife fitness, this chapter has addressed three vital components of your exercise program: aerobic exercise, strength training exercise, and weight-bearing exercise. The most intelligent way to exercise is to combine all three components and evaluate your exercise program by how much of your body you are using. For example, walking is weight-bearing but uses mostly your lower body, so by adding strength training for the upper body you'll achieve total body fitness.

Swimming isn't weight-bearing but does use your upper body, so by adding lower body strength training on other days, you'll cover all three components. Another option is choosing an activity that targets your fat cells, muscles, and bones simultaneously such as cross-country skiing outdoors or backpacking in the mountains.

In summary, to get the most out of your exercise program, combine aerobics, strength training, and weight-bearing activities, but don't go overboard. Pace yourself. In addition, you can also incorporate some of these tricks of the fitness trade:

- **Manage seemingly impossible schedules by practicing time-sensitive fitness.** Use ankle weights while you're walking around the house or making dinner, use wrist weights while you're cleaning the house, take the stairs instead of the elevator, carry the grocery bag instead of carting it to your car, take a walk in the airport during layovers, walk to an appointment instead of taking a cab or driving, keep an extra set of weights in your office to pull out when you have a few minutes, say "yes" when your child or grandchild asks for a piggyback ride. The possibilities are endless.

- **Do your mental workout before your physical workout.** Relax, center yourself, find your alignment, and mentally prepare yourself to exercise.

- **Get into a rhythm.** Repetitive movements can put you into a meditative state and make the time fly by.

- **Listen to music.** You'll automatically exercise 25 percent longer without realizing it. Wash the car to "Working at the Car Wash" by the Pointer Sisters, stack wood to Chopin, garden to Vivaldi's *Four Seasons*, or walk to "These Boots Are Made for Walking" by Nancy Sinatra.

- **Focus on your breathing.** We breathe over 25,000 times a day, but we seldom take full, deep breaths when we exercise. Oxygen is needed for the release of fat, so breathe deeply and let the oxygen flow.

- **Practice what's being called the "Tao of Training."**
  Visualize your muscles contracting and your fat cells releasing fat, imagine a calming place like the ocean, and connect with your energy to achieve exercise enlightenment.

There are new classes across the country where the instructors recite Buddhist readings while you're peddling on a stationary bike. There are also health clubs where you can stare at a screen of the ocean while you're on the rowing machine or a tape of the Himalayan mountains when you're walking on the treadmill.

Maybe not for you, but the message is that exercise should be relaxing, calming, and unstressful. That's why yoga and T'ai Chi are becoming more and more popular. By holding various poses, these exercises strengthen your muscles without stressing you out. You don't have to view exercise as work, one more obligation to beat yourself up about and wind up leaving the gym more stressed than when you entered.

Instead of going for the burn, pushing yourself to the limit, calculating your heart rate, and competing with others and yourself—go for the balance, push yourself into a reflective state, and have fun.

HOW ABOUT A LITTLE FLOOR PLAY?

I always enjoy a good play on words—and why not some "floor play"? Kids are more fit when they play. Play is good for the body and good for the soul. Get down on the floor with a child and anything can happen.

When we think of floor exercises, we automatically think of sit-ups, leg lifts, and push-ups. But when was the last time you got down on the floor and did a somersault, a leap frog, or a cartwheel? When was the last time that you got out on the dance floor and spent a couple of hours swinging, bumping, or two-stepping?

Thousands of women are trading in their aerobic shoes for tap shoes. Dance is so much more than a workout; it's also cultural and expressive. Many health clubs now offer dance-oriented classes such as hip-hop, cardiogroove, funk, and jazz. And dance studios have always offered ballet, modern dance, belly dance, African dance, Brazilian dance, Irish dance, tap dance, and square dance, to mention only a few. Or, a simpler option is to put on your favorite music, close the curtains if you must, make up your own routine, and dance the fat away.

The floor is great for playing, dancing, and stretching. Stretching is a component of fitness that is often overlooked. As we grow older, muscles and tendons shorten, so stretching for a few minutes during your warm-up and after your workout becomes even more important. By taking the time to stretch, you'll have less injury, fewer back problems, and greater mobility. Yoga is one of the best forms of stretching because it increases flexibility, balance, posture, and coordination.

To come back full circle—for all those times you always meant to exercise, now you will! But you'll do it with the knowledge that your midlife body is depending on it. And you'll do it with the enjoyment and passion that may have been lacking before. For all you may be experiencing during menopause, fitness will help bring your body back into a healthier balance. It's your menopausal stabilizer.

If you've gained fat, you can lose it,

if you've lost muscle, you can rebuild it,

if you've lost strength, you can regain it,

if you've lost bone mass, you can reverse it,

if you've lost energy, you can find it,

if you've lost sleep, you can catch up on it,

all through meno-positive fitness.

Find your internal motivator, set aside the time, pace yourself, enjoy yourself, and see what happens. The outcome may surprise you. It certainly surprised Kristen, who never thought she'd become a fitness convert. "I can't believe it. I want to do everything now: white-water raft, rollerblade, mountain climb, scuba dive, cross-country ski, do my own gardening, take karate lessons, wash my own car. I'm even planning a skydiving jump for next month."

You may not have quite the same transformation as Kristen, but I guarantee you that fitness will change your life forever.

HOW WILL YOU MASTER MENO-POSITIVE FITNESS?

I hope that I have presented a convincing argument for making exercise a priority during your midlife years. Now, it's time either to start exercising or to tailor your current program specifically for menopause. Check all of the following that make sense, feel right, and feel good to you, and you'll be on your way to mastering meno-positive fitness:

❏ I will release any guilt about not having exercised.

❏ I will acknowledge the benefits of fitness that are important to me.

❏ I will consider exercise a priority and make the time to do it.

❏ I will find my internal motivators.

❏ I will pace myself and start slowly.

❏ I will design an exercise program that's right for my personality and lifestyle.

❏ I will consult with my doctor before starting an exercise program

❏ I will progressively add aerobic activity and work up to four hours a week to release fat.

❏ I will monitor my heart rate, rate of breathing, and never feel out of breath.

❏ I will progressively add strength-training activities and work up to one hour a week to build my 639 muscles.

❏ I will consult an exercise physiologist or certified personal trainer if I need assistance with my strength-training program.

❏ I will include some weight-bearing exercises each week.

❏ I will not overexercise.

❏ I will evaluate my exercise program by how much muscle mass I am using.

❏ I will do my mental workout before my physical workout.

❏ I will get into a rhythm and pay attention to my breathing.

❏ I will stretch during my warm-up and after my workout.

❏ I will listen to music.

❏ I will have fun.

❏ I will take the next step of embracing meno-positive eating habits by reading the next chapter.

chapter six

EMBRACING
MENO-POSITIVE
EATING HABITS

Picture one of your midlife fat cells: It's round, probably still larger than you'd like, and has two distinct sides that function independently of each other. The right side is responsible for the release of fat while the left side is busy working at storage. You've effectively mastered the right-hand side by manufacturing the fat-releasing enzymes with meno-positive fitness, but the left side has thus far been ignored.

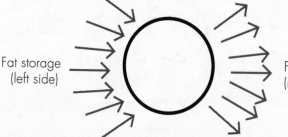

Fat storage
(left side)

Fat release
(right side)

If you stop reading this book right now, you will have only accomplished half of The Meno-Positive Approach and half of what it takes to outsmart your midlife fat cells. Your fat cells will be releasing with exercise, but they will also still be storing with your eating habits. And storage is high on the list of menopausal fat cell priorities.

You have more storage enzymes today than you had as a premenopausal woman, which makes you 20 percent more efficient in taking every little extra calorie, scooping it up, and storing it in your fat cells (especially those at your waist). Coupled with more storage power, your metabolism is also 10 to 15 percent lower than it was a few years ago. So, not only are you more efficient at storage, you also have more surplus to store. Specifically, at least 300 more calories to store each day and 100,000 to store over a year!

But don't panic! We're now going to shift gears and turn our attention to the left side of your fat cells to deactivate this storage. When you embrace meno-positive eating habits, all systems will work to store less, release more, and shrink your fat cells permanently—and both the left and right sides of your fat cells will be working in tandem to make you leaner. Soon, your fat cells will look like this:

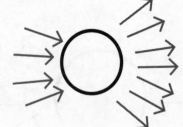

Embracing
meno-positive
eating habits

Mastering
meno-positive
fitness

How meno-positive are your eating habits? When I ask new clients to tell me about their eating habits, they usually begin by defending their food choices. "I don't eat much fat, I stay away from sugar, and I buy mostly low calorie foods. How can I be gaining weight even though I'm eating healthier?"

Because there's more to our eating habits than healthy food choices. What we eat is only a relatively small part of the weight gain (or weight loss) equation. This comes as a surprise to many women because of the "you are what you eat" philosophy that governs our society. Because we have been taught that if you eat less fat, you'll weigh less, reducing fat intake is our number one dietary goal. Three-quarters of us report that we are eating less fat, but paradoxically, few report that fat reduction has led to weight reduction. In fact, most report that their weights have somehow climbed higher with a low-fat diet.

The reason for this puzzling weight gain is that we're overeating reduced-fat foods. ***It's not "you are <u>what</u> you eat";*** ***it's "you are <u>how much</u> you eat."***

We all know what to eat: less fat, more fruits and vegetables, more fiber, more variety. But we no longer know how much to eat. We don't know how to eat moderately.

I'll teach you how. At first, you may feel frustrated that I'm not addressing actual food choices. You may want to know "But what should I be eating?" I'll answer that question in the next chapter. For now, eat what you want and concentrate on:

- **why** you're eating
- **when** you're eating, and
- **how much** you're eating

Perhaps you've already heard some of what I'm going to suggest before: eat when you're hungry; eat smaller, more frequent meals; and eat less at night. Maybe you've even followed some of these recommendations before. But this time you're going to hear and adhere to them as they apply to your changing midlife body.

Before you begin, reflect on your current eating habits by answering the following questions:

		yes	no
1.	Do you often ignore your hunger signals?	_____	_____
2.	Do you often skip meals?	_____	_____
3.	Do you regularly feel full after you eat?	_____	_____
4.	Do you avoid snacking?	_____	_____
5.	Is dinner your largest meal of the day?	_____	_____
6.	Do you often snack after dinner?	_____	_____
7.	Do you often feel guilty after eating?	_____	_____
8.	Are you usually starving by suppertime?	_____	_____
9.	Do you eat by the clock?	_____	_____
10.	Do you eat to distract yourself from uncomfortable emotions?	_____	_____
11.	Do you eat to reward yourself after a hard day?	_____	_____
12.	Do you freely eat "good" foods but deprive yourself of "bad" ones?	_____	_____

If many, most, or all of these habits describe your eating behavior, then you have much to gain from the information that follows—and you are not alone. According to a recent survey by the American Dietetic Association, 66 percent of adult women say that they select foods based on "good" and "bad" evaluations, 50 percent say that their eating experiences are void of pleasure, and 36 percent say that they feel guilty after eating the foods they like. Bad, pleasureless, guilt-ridden—that's how too many of us feel about eating.

You may have spent the last thirty years having negative

feelings about food, but with this chapter, you'll spend the next thirty years feeling positive about your eating.

TAP INTO YOUR BODY OF KNOWLEDGE

Somewhere, deep down, buried below the layers of dieting, guilt, and society's eating rules, you have all the knowledge and wisdom to embrace meno-positive eating habits on your own. You have the instincts to eat in a way that's right for your body and to lose any excess weight. You were born with these instincts—and they can't wait for their rebirth.

You may think that someone else knows better than you about how you're supposed to eat—that a health professional, homeopathic healer, writer, talk show host, health food store employee, diet counselor, friend, or celebrity has the know-how to teach you how to eat. They don't. You may think that a diet plan has the ability to teach you healthy eating habits. It doesn't. Every single diet you've ever followed is based on the assumption that you lack intelligence when it comes to eating—when in fact, you're the only one who has the smarts. I'll prove to you that you have them, show you how to recognize your eating instincts, and teach you how to tap into your body's food wisdom.

If society's eating rules didn't exist and dieting was never invented, how do you think you would naturally eat? Here's how Diane answered this question: "I would eat whenever and wherever I wanted to, I wouldn't worry so much about sugar and fat, and I would nibble all day long and forgo meals entirely."

Bingo! This was how Diane's body would instinctively direct her eating for health, vitality, and well-being, and how she would outsmart her menopausal fat cells. She didn't believe me at first either (I'm assuming you're skeptical too) until she pretended that she lived in a nonjudgmental utopia where there was no right or wrong way of eating. For three months, she ate when her body told her to eat, responded to hunger instead of the clock, nibbled on moderate amounts, and ended up eating about eight times a day. Over those three months, she felt her body change and discovered that she had lost almost 2 percent of her body fat (P.S. she was also exercising five hours a week with aerobics and strength training).

You may find that eating eight times a day is not instinctive eating for you, but five times a day is. Each of us is different, with varying metabolisms and food needs. However, several eating instincts are common to most menopausal women because our bodies are going through the same unique changes.

EATING INSTINCT	BIOLOGICAL REASON
eat frequently	menopausal women are more sensitive to changes in blood sugar levels; eating every few hours keeps blood sugar stable and energy high throughout the day
snack often	for the same reasons as above and for an extra boost of energy and more stable moods
eat our largest meal at lunch	metabolism and caloric needs are highest midday
eat our smallest meal at dinner	during midlife, our metabolism takes a nose dive at 6 P.M., and caloric needs become almost nonexistent at night
eat smaller amounts overall	our bodies need 200 to 400 fewer calories a day and will automatically adjust to this lower calorie level by requiring a little less food at each meal

How many of these instincts do you naturally follow? One of my clients answered, "Not one. Actually, this is the direct opposite of the way I've been eating all of my adult life. I've been skipping meals, staying away from snacking, eating next to nothing for lunch, and devouring several platefuls at dinner. I think my eating instincts jumped ship in 1980 and are lost at sea."

There's no question that this woman and you have natural eating instincts, the question is, How are you going to find them and bring them to the surface? The answer is, **Go on a hunger hunt.**

Your eating instincts are located in your brain, body, and stomach and are communicated to you via feelings of hunger. How does your body signal hunger?

- Does it originate in your stomach? With growls, pangs, and churning?

- Does it originate in your brain? With fogginess, lack of concentration, and headaches?

- Does it originate in your body? With an overall lack of energy?

Hunger is the *only* way your body can inform you that it needs to be refueled. Trust your body's hunger signals; they will tell you when to eat. As you're making the decision to eat, check in with your hunger—and you'll know what to do.

- If you're hungry, you'll know that your body needs fuel, and you'll benefit from eating by having more energy, more stable moods, and greater productivity. Your fat cells are not a beneficiary of responding to hunger; the calories will be burned up by your body before your fat cells ever get a chance to store.

- If you're not hungry, you'll know that your body doesn't need food, and there's no benefit to eating, except to your fat cells, which will profit greatly from storage.

When Ilene checked in with her stomach to see if it was communicating hunger, she reported, "My stomach's ignoring me. It's not returning my phone calls." If you check in and never get past a dial tone, maybe it's because you've been ignoring your hunger for years, quelling it with diet soft drinks and coffee or following restrictive diets. Any liquid will temporarily fill your stomach, and any diet will disconnect your hunger signals.

With dieting, you're instructed to eat a specific amount of food at a predetermined time. Hunger is ignored, and eventually, your body gives up on you and stops sending hunger signals. You haven't responded for years, so why bother expending the energy to transmit the message? It's a two-way street: You need to trust your body's hunger signals, and your body needs to trust that you'll respond to them. Give your body time to start trusting you again. Once you yield to your hunger, the other instinctive eating habits will follow.

As you begin tapping into your body of knowledge, perhaps some of the ways my clients have reconnected to their own hunger signals will give you some ideas:

- Simone started with just one meal. She wouldn't commit to eating every time she was hungry, but she did agree to wait until she was hungry before eating her next meal. She felt hungry, ate, and found the experience interesting enough to want to do it again. As she said, "Hunger was a surprisingly pleasant sensation, not at all uncomfortable like I thought it would be."

- Lucy asked herself "Am I hungry?" every time she was about to put food into her mouth. This kept her connected to her body's food needs with a simple "yes" or "no" answer.

- Jane thought of her stomach as a gas tank and her hunger as a fuel gauge. When she "read" her hunger, she would assess whether her stomach was half empty, three quarters empty, or in the red zone warning her that she had to refuel soon or she would completely run out of gas.

- Patricia, a veterinarian, made a game out of it. She used animals to categorize her hunger signals: Was she hungry as a bird, a horse, or a lion with the loudest, most powerful stomach growl?

- At first, Jeri didn't experience hunger, so she followed the general recommendation to make sure she ate something small every three to four hours. Within two weeks, her body got used to being fed small amounts every few hours, and she reported feeling hunger for the first time in ten years.

And by the way, all of these women lost body fat. You, too, can choose to lose by listening to your hunger. ***Ignore and you'll store.***

Here's what happens if you ignore your hunger signals and don't eat when you're hungry: Within thirty minutes your body starts to wonder what's going on and intensifies its hunger signals to try to get your attention. After another thirty minutes your body starts to get nervous that it may never get food: Is something wrong? Are you incapable of eating? Is food unavailable? And your foolproof survival mechanism kicks into gear by slowing down your metabolism, breaking down your muscle mass and carbohydrate stores, stimulating your fat-storage enzymes, and disconnecting your hunger signals. Haven't you noticed how ravenous hunger miraculously goes away when enough time has passed? One of my clients thought disappearing hunger was a sign that her calorie needs were satisfied by her fat cells releasing fat. Wishful thinking. She was disappointed to hear that fat stores don't release with hunger; glucose and muscle stores do. Instead, the fat cells recruit extra forces, stimulate more fat-storage enzymes, and get ready for the truckload of food when your hunger comes back full force.

NEITHER STARVE NOR STUFF

When you diet, fast, skip meals, or ignore your hunger for hours, your body will do everything it possibly can to get you to eat—and eat a lot.

- Your salivation increases so that mouth-watering foods are even more irresistible.

- A potent chemical, neuropeptide Y, is released to increase your desire for carbohydrates—your body's primary and preferred energy source.

- Another equally persuasive chemical, galanin, is released to increase your craving for fat—the quickest way to get plenty of calories into your starving body.

- The appetite center in your brain is stimulated so that any food will do (carbohydrate, fat, or protein), whether you like the food or not.

The powerful result of this biological starvation response: eat a lot, eat it quickly, then eat some more just to play it safe. First we starve, then we stuff—*not because **we** lack control, but because **our bodies** are in complete control.*

Undereating causes overeating. Self-imposed famines cause self-destructive feasts. For every period of food deprivation, your body makes sure there is an equal and opposite binge. Every time you've gone on a diet you've experienced this starvation response, and every time you've skipped a meal you've experienced it. When was the last time your eating was influenced by this starve-stuff phenomenon?

For Sarah, it was yesterday and every day before that. Sarah is a meal skipper, with lunch being the neglected meal of choice. By late afternoon, she found she was so ravenous that she would devour massive amounts standing up at the kitchen counter. Her body forced her to overeat to make up for what she should have eaten hours ago at lunch when her body was hungry. At the end of her eating frenzy, feeling stuffed and fearing weight gain, she vowed to skip lunch again the next day. Her undereating during the day caused overeating at night, which in turn caused undereating the next day.

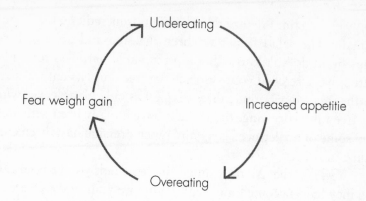

Because of this strong cause-and-effect relationship, many women's eating habits vacillate between starving and stuffing. Some women deprive and binge daily. Others undereat during the week and then overeat on the weekends. And all women deprive their bodies when they diet and then overindulge for weeks after the diet is over. No wonder we are gaining more weight than we need to during perimenopause. We are unknowingly helping our fat cells expand with undereating and overeating.

Whenever you overeat and feel full, the stretch receptors on the wall of your stomach send a message to your brain that a substantial amount of food was just consumed. This is all the information your brain gets. It doesn't know exactly what has filled your stomach to capacity, it only knows that the gauge registers full. So with this limited information, your brain in turn sends a message to your fat cells to activate their fat-storage enzymes and get ready to work (needless to say, your fat cells are ecstatic with this news).

This stomach-to-brain communication happens when you eat a heaping plate of pasta, a few extra pieces of pizza, a triple-decker sandwich, a twelve-ounce steak, or a massive salad with nonfat dressing. A nonfat salad? You can bet on it. Overeating a nonfat, low-calorie food such as a salad can lead to fat storage and weight gain. I realize that this sounds incredible, but let me explain. The salad hasn't yet been digested and absorbed, so your brain doesn't know that a presumably harmless food like lettuce has stretched your stomach to three times its natural size. By the time your brain realizes that it was only plant leaves with fat-free ranch dressing, the fat cells have already been activated and some of the lettuce leaves and ranch dressing have been corralled into your waist.

Yes, it's true. All those huge fat-free salads you've been eating may have become fat once they got into your body. Overeating is overeating. Of course the salads would have to be massive to cause fat storage, but it's best to work with the premise that overeating *anything* can lead to weight gain. And because your menopausal body is actively storing fat twenty-four hours a day anyway to produce estrogen, this also means that you are a superefficient fat-free cookie storer, rice cake storer, carrot storer, and nonfat frozen yogurt storer too.

I share this shocking news about fat storage to reinforce the point that **what you eat is not as important as how much you eat.** The second most effective way to outsmart your midlife fat cells (if your memory needs jogging, go jogging—the first was exercise) is to **fill your stomach without overfilling it.**

Do you know the difference between filling your stomach and overfilling it? Do you know the difference between feeling satisfied and feeling uncomfortably full? These distinctions may help:

FILLING YOUR STOMACH	OVERFILLING IT
You feel no change in the way your clothes fit.	Your waistband is noticeably tighter; unbuttoning the top button of your pants is a telltale sign.

When you look at your profile in the mirror, you see no extension of your stomach.	You see so much extension that you're reminded of pregnancy.
If you really wanted to, you could go out for a walk right after eating.	You barely have the energy to get up from the table.
You get hungry again in another three to four hours.	Your stomach is so full that it takes six to eight hours of labored digestion before you get hungry again.

Now for another important question: Do you know how much food it takes for you to fill your stomach without overfilling it? If you turn to Miss Piggy for advice, she says, "Never eat more than you can lift." My guess is that Miss Piggy is not an instinctive eater, so let's revise that to **"Never eat more than you can lift with one hand."**

Believe it or not, your stomach is about the size of your fist. To prevent overexpansion and fat storage, a good-size handful of food will fill your stomach adequately without overfilling it. Chewing decreases the volume of food, so a handful becomes a fistful by the time it reaches your stomach.

How much do you usually eat? Is it a handful? A plateful? A bagful? A boxful? A bowlful? Let's do an experiment. Get up, go into the kitchen, and get a bag of popcorn (or chips or pretzels). Pour into a bowl the amount you normally eat, then pour the bowl into the palm of your hand. Where's most of the popcorn? Is it in your hand or on the countertop?

When Terry did this experiment, she discovered that she was eating three times what her body needed. She also turned this experiment into her anti-overeating strategy by making it a usual practice to use her hand to measure out food. Her family thought she was a bit unusual, but at the beginning, it guaranteed that she wasn't overeating.

You don't have to start measuring out handfuls of food, but

you can visually assess by asking "How much of this meal or snack will fit into my hand?" It may be half of the sandwich instead of the whole one, a third of your plate of pasta, three-quarters of your lasagna, or the whole bowl of ice cream.

The next time you are tempted by an extra handful or another helping of anything:

- **Take a tummy time-out.** Get up from the table and take five minutes to give your body a chance to tell you that it's satisfied. If you keep eating, your body may have been ready to tell you to stop, but the mouthfuls just kept coming, and your body had to divert its attention to storage.

- **Go into the bathroom and brush your teeth to finalize eating.** Food never tastes as good right after you brush your teeth.

- **Visualize that extra food feeding your fat cells.** With fork, knife, and napkin in ready position, think of your fat cells gobbling up their feast and wish them "bon appetit."

- **Tell yourself that you can have another helping in a few hours when your body tells you it's hungry again.** You're better off eating more later than eating everything all at once.

- **Do everything you can to prevent being overhungry _before_ you start eating.** It's much easier to eat moderately when your body isn't in a starvation state. Your appetite center isn't working overtime and your body isn't forcing you to overeat. Make sure you quickly respond to your hunger signals, eating whenever you're hungry—and I mean whenever. Have a few crackers when you're in line at the post office, when you're waiting for the bus, when you're in a meeting, and when you're driving to an appointment.

- **Record how much you're eating and how your body feels after eating.** Many of us think we are not eating much until we see it down on paper. If I asked you to recite everything you ate yesterday, chances are you would "forget" at least a third of your intake. And your amnesia would be selective. You'd remember every vegetable and piece of fruit, but forget the candy bar, chips, and peanuts.

If these strategies don't work, and you've just got to have that second helping—be aware of what you're doing, make a conscious decision to overeat, and don't worry. You'll be happy to hear that overeating every now and then will not cause any storage and may actually be advantageous. In fact, I actually "prescribe" occasional overeating to a handful of clients.

When overeating is a predictable event because it happens all the time, your brain says, "Here we go again, way too much food. Fat cells, you know the score, so hurry up and store." But when it happens on rare occasions, your brain says, "What's going on here! Where did all this food come from? What on earth am I going to do with it?" In a panic, your brain activates every possible way to get rid of the excess calories. It stimulates your muscle mass to use more, your metabolism to burn more, and your fat cells to store more. But, by the time the calories get to the fat cells, most of them have already been disposed of. Occasional overeating teaches your midlife body that there are alternatives to storage.

When you tap into your body of knowledge, listen to your body's signals of hunger, neither starve nor stuff, and seldom overeat—you'll find that you'll automatically eat smaller meals, more snacks, more food during the day, and less food at night.

DOWNSIZE YOUR MEALS, UPGRADE YOUR SNACKING

Breakfast foods aren't just for breakfast anymore. Sandwiches aren't just for lunch anymore. Meat and potatoes aren't just for dinner anymore. Snacking isn't just for kids anymore. When you become an instinctive eater, you'll be breaking all the eating rules.

The truth is, **Midlife women need to eat midmorning, midday, and midafternoon.** We need to double the number of times we eat throughout the day with more meals and snacks.

The typical perimenopausal woman eats two and a half times a day—half of what our bodies and brains require for optimal functioning. Eating five or more times a day provides a steady and dependable source of glucose to our brains, balancing our mood swings and boosting our energy. Studies have shown that when midlife women let more than four hours pass between meals, many of the troublesome signs intensify: anxiety, depression, fatigue, memory loss, and confusion.

How many hours ago did you last eat? How do you feel right now? If it was less than four hours, I'd expect to hear a relatively positive report. If it was more than four hours, you may be having a difficult time comprehending this paragraph because your brain is lacking the glucose it needs to concentrate. Take a break; you're hungry. Go get something to eat and come back rejuvenated.

If you're not eating at least five times a day, most likely it's because you're avoiding snacks and skipping meals. Which meal do you think women are most likely to skip? The answer is the most important one—lunch. Mississippi State University found that lunch was skipped most often and dinner was skipped least often (the only meal we should consider skipping every now and then). We need to upgrade our daytime meals and snacks, and downgrade our dinners. In other words, *we need to focus on matching our eating to our new menopausal metabolism.*

Everyone's metabolism is highest during the first twelve hours of the day and lowest during the second twelve hours of the day, but menopausal women have a 10 to 15 percent lower metabolism all day long and a 10 to 15 percent bigger drop in metabolism at night.

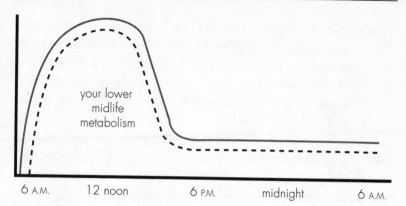

your lower
midlife
metabolism

6 A.M.   12 noon   6 P.M.   midnight   6 A.M.

It's easy to match your eating to your metabolism at break-fast. We seldom overeat breakfast, and the typical breakfast rarely reaches 500 calories. This is why I recommended eating breakfast at any time of the day. At lunch, we consume about 500 calories (and could stand to eat even a few hundred calories more). But at dinner, we top 1,000 calories! Your body doesn't need the 1,000 calories at night. Where do they go? By now you know the answer all too well—directly to your fat cells. Night-time eating means partytime for your fat cells.

As a friend of mine has always said, "Eat a hearty breakfast with your family, share lunch with a friend, and give dinner away to an enemy." If you have someone particular in mind, bring out a five-course dinner every night, and it won't take long to get your retribution.

For you, your family, and your friends, add something else to this sound advice: provide a ready supply of snacks for your body all day long. Snacking when you're hungry doesn't cause weight gain; it promotes weight loss. It prevents you from overeating at meals and helps you eat less overall. But snack se-riously—make it count, eat a variety of different foods, think of it as a minimeal, and use a handful to determine how much to eat.

With both snacks and meals, we are usually better at utilizing the handful maneuver at home, but as soon as we leave the house, our hands are solely used to finish the package or clean our plates. Because meals eaten away from home account for one-third of our food intake, we have to learn how to bring instinctive eating to the restaurant and the snack counter.

Everywhere we look there are king-size candy bars, Big Gulp soft drinks, Big Foot pizzas, foot long hot dogs, supersize French fries, family-size packages (that are often eaten with no help from the family), and all-you-can-eat buffets. In fact, we're the only country in the world with these jumbo size products, and the only people who seek out the "all-you-can-eat for $8.99" establishments. These products and buffets seem normal to us, but other societies are perplexed with our strange eating behavior.

Economically, we say the larger products and meals are a better buy. We get more for our investment, but most of the food is being banked in our fat cells as we strive to get our money's worth. Larger plates and packages lead to larger bodies. We all need to become educated on portion sizes, including health professionals. A recent study asked dietitians to estimate the calorie content of various portions served at restaurants, and on average, they underestimated by 50 percent! If *we* can't do it and are inadvertently eating more than we need at restaurants, how can we expect *you* to?

The Center for Science in the Public Interest recently did an eye-opening analysis of various away-from-home foods and found that restaurant serving sizes were two to eight times larger than the standard serving sizes recommended by the USDA.

	RESTAURANT SERVING	STANDARD SERVING
McDonald's SuperSize French fries	6 oz. 540 cal	3 oz. 220 cal
movie theater popcorn (medium)	16 cups 900 cal	3 cups 160 cal
tuna sandwich	⅔ lb. 720 cal	¼ lb. 340 cal
7-Eleven Double Gulp Soda	64 oz. 800 cal	8 oz. 100 cal
muffin	4 oz. 430 cal	2 oz. 190 cal
spaghetti with tomato sauce	3½ cups 850 cal	1 cup 250 cal

One of the biggest shockers is the steak comparison. A typical three-ounce serving of steak has only 170 calories, but a steak house serving is close to a pound and has 1,150 calories!

Whether at home, at work, or at a restaurant, be aware of how much you're eating. When you start eating smaller meals and more snacks, you'll want to continue with this routine because your stomach will shrink in size. Your stomach is like a balloon and within a couple of weeks of decreasing meal size, you'll need less food to fill it up. Columbia University researchers found that when people ate larger meals, their stomachs grew larger and it took progressively more food to satisfy their hunger. When people were given smaller meals, stomach capacity decreased by one-third, and they progressively ate less.

Eating smaller meals and decreasing stomach capacity can be difficult when you have young children at home and value the importance of family meals. You can still have this meaningful family time, just put a smaller amount on *your* plate.

Another obstacle to eating smaller meals is emotional eating. Menopausal women have heightened emotions, and during the transition, loneliness, depression, anxiety, fatigue, and mood swings may seem unbearable, and food may be sought for solace.

EMOTIONAL EATING VS. EATING EMOTIONALLY

Do you know the difference between physical hunger and emotional hunger?

Physical hunger is when your body needs nourishment.

Emotional hunger is when your soul needs nourishment.

Any confusion between the two could have begun many years ago. As a child, you may have been given a treat to provide comfort during painful times. You may have watched your mother turn to the kitchen when she was upset or sad. Or the blur between physical and emotional hunger could be a more recent confusion that began after a divorce, a layoff, or other difficult event. We often turn to food because it distracts us; we forget the pain for a while, the blood rushes from the brain to the stomach for digestion, and we feel numb. Many of us eat to fight fatigue, depression, and stress—battles that can never be won with food.

Instead of using food (an unsuccessful, external weapon) to cope with emotions, turn inward. We are more in tune with our bodies and minds during menopause and, therefore, can use this opportunity to more accurately identify our emotions, then give ourselves what we really need to nourish our souls. These tried and true questions will help you in this process:

What am I feeling?
What do I really need?

When you specifically identify what you are feeling, maybe you'll find what you really need is a good cry, a good laugh, a good bath, a good run, a good nap . . . a good therapist? Licensed therapists have the skills to help you express your feelings in a safe environment and take care of your emotional needs in a nonfood way.

If distraction from your feelings is what you're after, do something other than eating that will accomplish this goal: get engrossed in a page-turning book, rent a tear-jerking movie, clean out your closet (or come over to my house and clean out mine), take a drive to the beach or the mountains, take a long nap, or get together with a good friend to talk. Acknowledge what you are doing and why, identify your feelings, and realize that food is the last thing you need.

When I asked Carmen whether or not she thought she was an emotional eater, she excitedly replied, "Oh, most definitely! My whole family is. We talk about food all the time, plan delicious meals together, and share recipes. Every dish is prepared emotionally, and every meal is eaten emotionally. We spend hours at the dinner table laughing, singing, telling jokes, and enjoying our meals. We eat very emotionally."

I loved Carmen's answer. Of course, she and her family were not emotional eaters in the clinical sense of using food to fulfill emotional needs; they simply ate emotionally, which I strongly advocate.

Eating emotionally is eating with passion, experiencing the pleasure, satisfaction, and enjoyment with every bite. The French eat emotionally. They consume many high-fat and high-cholesterol foods, but they don't carry the extra weight or have the high heart disease risk that we do. Feeling emotional about food is healthy. It gives us more satisfaction with the whole experience of eating and, therefore, helps us to eat less, and weigh less.

Eating affects us all on an emotional level. It's exciting to go out to our favorite restaurant. It's comforting to eat a hot food on a cold day. It's special for me to receive mashed potatoes and gravy from my mother every time I go home to Maine for a visit. It's fun to eat cake on our birthday. Yet many of us have forgotten how to eat emotionally and have fun with food.

If you were to have uninhibited fun with food, what would you do? Specifically, what would you do with m&m's? Would you line them up before eating them? Eat them by color? Bite them in half first? Try to pry the shell off? Try to get them to melt in your hands? The next time you eat m&m's, put some in the palm of your hand, play with them, and eat them slowly. You'll discover that a handful (instead of a bagful) is all you need to feel wonderfully satisfied.

IT'S MIND OVER PLATTER

Let's assume you're visiting a friend, and she places a plate of cheese and crackers in front of you. If you're hungry, you can choose to eat a handful. Or, if you don't like cheese and crackers, you can ask for something else. Or, if you're not hungry, you can choose to listen to your body telling you it has no need for food at this moment. You might move a little farther away from the plate or tell your friend that you're not hungry right now.

This would be an example of "mind over platter," tapping into your body of knowledge and eating instinctively. The plate of cheese and crackers doesn't control you; you control the plate. You're the decision maker—choosing whether or not you eat and how much you eat.

There are pioneers and newcomers to this internal approach. Jane Hirschmann and Carol Munter paved the way by calling it Demand Feeding in their book, *Overcoming Overeating*. Susan Kano called it Spontaneous Eating in her book, *Making Peace with Food*. In Evelyn Tribole and Elyse Resch's book, *Intuitive Eating*, the title speaks for itself, telling us to use our intuition to direct our food choices.

I have called it *instinctive eating* throughout this and my other books. Regardless of what we call the internal approach, the rules are the same: *there are no rules*. There are no plans to follow, no guidelines to adhere to, and no standard behavior modification techniques to employ. Rules, techniques, and plans are instructions coming from the outside instead of instincts originating from the inside. That's why behavior modification techniques such as using a smaller plate, not reading or watching TV while eating, taking twenty minutes to eat a meal, and putting your fork down between each bite may not be helpful

Behavior modification is often just a fancy term for "rules," and rules are meant to be broken. I break them all the time. I sometimes eat while watching TV, I use a regular-size plate, and I don't always take twenty minutes to eat, yet I know that I eat instinctively.

Regardless of what you're doing or what size plate you're using, your menopausal body can effectively direct your eating. Even if you've been eating instinctively for many years, your instincts are now changing because your body is changing. As a premenopausal woman, four small meals a day may have kept your fat cells in check, but now six minimeals may be necessary to outsmart them. Snacking may have been important to you then, but now because your moods are more volatile, it's critical. The changes in your eating instincts may be subtle or significant, but they are your midlife solution to achieving a fit, healthy body.

You just have to stay connected to your hunger and your body's food needs. Sit for a moment before you eat to take inventory of your hunger and take in the visual sensation of the plate of food. Pause while you eat to enjoy the taste and prevent feeling full. And sit after you eat to make the experience last. Think of each meal as a work of art—admire it, appreciate it, use all your senses, and treasure the pleasure.

If you could artfully design your next meal as the plate of your dreams, what would it be?

Even if it's fettuccini Alfredo, I say excellent! A fine plate of your dreams. Mine is double-cut lamb chops with garlic mashed potatoes. Whatever it is, don't be too concerned about the fat, sugar, or calorie content. Instead, focus on eating it instinctively with the following suggestions. First, make sure you're hungry when you eat it. Next, eat one-quarter of it, pause, and check in with your body: Is it happy? Are you happy? Are you satisfied? Have you eaten enough to satisfy your hunger? If the answer is no, then eat another quarter of it and repeat the questions. When you've eaten enough to satisfy your hunger without overeating, rest assured that none of the calories or fat will be stored in your fat cells—and just think of the delicious leftovers you'll have to-morrow!

HOW WILL YOU EMBRACE MENO-POSITIVE EATING HABITS?

Look at how far you've come. You've made the decision to work with your menopausal fat cells instead of against them. You've made the decision to make exercise a part of your life and master meno-positive fitness. Now you're about to decide how you are going to change your eating habits to become an instinctive eater. Check all of the following that make sense, feel right, and feel good to you, and you'll be on your way to embracing meno-positive eating habits:

❑ I will evaluate my eating habits by *how much* I'm eating, not *what* I'm eating.

❑ I will tap into my body's instinctive eating wisdom.

❑ I will discover how my body communicates hunger and respond to its signals.

❑ I will ask myself "Am I hungry?" before I start eating.

❑ I will neither starve nor stuff.

❑ I will not deny my body food when I'm hungry.

❑ I will fill my stomach without overfilling it.

❑ I will realize that fat-free foods can become stored fat if I overeat them.

❑ I will use a handful to estimate a moderate amount of food.

❑ I will take a tummy time-out by pausing while I'm eating to give my body a chance to tell me when it's had enough.

❑ I will consider it perfectly natural to overeat every now and then.

❑ I will permit myself to snack when I'm hungry.

❑ I will match my eating to my menopausal metabolism by eating more during the day and less at night.

❑ I will view lunch as my most important meal of the day.

❑ I will ask, "What am I feeling? What do I really need?" to identify my emotions and take care of myself in a nonfood way.

❑ I will eat emotionally—with passion, satisfaction, and enjoyment.

❑ I will have fun with food.

❑ I will eat the plate of my dreams.

❑ I will take the next step of maximizing meno-positive food choices by reading the next chapter.

chapter seven

MAXIMIZING
MENO-POSITIVE
FOOD CHOICES

f I told you to pile your plate high with lutein, indoles, and ly-copene; top it with bioflavonoids; toss it with linoleic acid; sip some phenols; and finish the meal with phenylethylamine covered anthocyanins—would you know what I was talking about?

I wouldn't necessarily expect you to, but lately it seems like the world of nutrition has gone warp speed into the future, bombarding us with space-age terms that make us feel as though we need a degree in biochemistry even to pronounce them. These attention-getting words are plant sources of powerful chemicals including estrogens, antioxidents, essential fatty acids, and other disease fighting substances. And these beneficial phytochemicals (*phyto* means plant), as they are called, are quickly making their way into the press and our vocabularies. What this paragraph really says is

Pile your plate high with spinach, broccoli, and tomatoes; top it with some tofu; toss it with full-fat salad dressing; sip some wine; and finish the meal with chocolate-covered strawberries.

Does that sound so bad? Some fat, chocolate, and wine (if you desire); some protein and a lot of vegetables and fruits. These foods and the benefits they offer are important to everyone regardless of age or gender, but they are especially important to *you* during menopause. As you'll discover, they enhance your well-being and smooth your transition while at the same time reducing your risk of disease.

You may be thinking that it's impossible for chocolate or high-fat salad dressing to be healthy food choices for menopause, but there are biological reasons for why chocolate may be a daily necessity instead of a craving to be given into monthly, why nonfat versions of foods are completely unsatisfying, and why vegetables are becoming more and more appealing. In fact, you may find that you are already eating more of these meno-positive foods because your body is naturally directing you to them. As a midlife woman, you have two factors working in your favor:

1. At age 35, virtually all women become more committed to healthy eating, and by age 55, we have the healthiest diets of all age groups with the highest intake of vegetables and fruits.

2. Women have an inborn food wisdom that keeps us connected to our changing nutritional needs, and during menopause, our bodies will guide us to eat those foods that will balance our bodies, stabilize our moods, and boost our energy.

Biologically, your body wants to eat in a way that's healthy for your midlife years, but psychologically, some obstacles may be preventing you from listening to your body's food wisdom and achieving a healthful diet. The top reasons cited for not eating more healthfully are:

• thinking we have to give up our favorite foods (like chocolate, ice cream, and chips) because they are "bad" for us—and we don't want to!

- feeling confused about the multitude of conflicting recommendations on what's healthy to eat

Some authorities say that we should emphasize carbohydrates in our diets; others say we should eliminate them. Some recommend a moderate amount of fat; others preach the evils of fat. Some label sugar as white death; others consider sugar a healthy food choice. It depends on who you ask or which magazine article or book you read. I call this "Food News Blues." Do you have it? I certainly do. It seems like every time we turn around, there's a contradictory report or study saying what we thought was healthy isn't. We don't know what to believe anymore!

What three-quarters of us do believe is that in the next five years experts will change their minds once again on what's healthy to eat. I happen to share this belief. How many of us switched from butter to margarine only to find out a few years later that margarine wasn't healthy either? How many gave up salt to later discover that in the majority of people salt was not linked to high blood pressure? How many resolved ourselves to a lifetime without eggs only to be recently told that we could eat four a week without affecting our heart disease risk? I could go on and on with examples, but the point is that if you feel frustrated and confused, that's a good sign. It means that your common sense is keeping things in perspective. **There are no concrete answers and no good or bad foods.**

My initial advice is to disregard most of the good food/bad food battle and listen to your common sense; it will tell you that a moderate amount of *any* food is healthy. Instead of focusing on what you shouldn't be eating, focus on what you should be eating. Fruits and vegetables have always been important; some fat, protein, and carbohydrates have always been necessary for health. According to an American Dietetic Association survey, over 60 percent of us want to do away with the negativism of doom-and-gloom nutrition and replace it with education on the positive aspects of food. In this chapter, I'll share the benefits of indulging in your favorite foods, the unmatched advantage of eating fruits and vegetables, and the value of including some fat, sugar, and chocolate in your diet. And with this knowledge, you'll confidently make your own positive food choices.

How meno-positive are your food choices right now? Take this very different quiz to find out.

1. Carrots are:
   a. a daily food choice
   b. only for making carrot cake
   c. only for rabbits

2. My plate usually consists of colors that are:
   a. a rainbow of brights
   b. pastels
   c. whites and browns

3. I'm more likely to cook with:
   a. a nonstick skillet
   b. a frying pan
   c. a deep fryer

4. Tofu is:
   a. a soy product
   b. a food found only in Japan
   c. a foot fungus

5. The last time I ate broccoli, Brussels sprouts, or spinach was:
   a. yesterday
   b. last week
   c. in grade school

6. My typical meat serving is as big as:
   a. a deck of cards

    b. a paperback novel

    c. a dictionary

7. I am more likely to keep water:

    a. by my side

    b. in my refrigerator

    c. in my carburetor

8. When I crave chocolate, I:

    a. happily eat some

    b. unhappily sneak some when no one is looking

    c. lock myself in the bathroom so I won't eat it

9. If there's something green on my plate, it's usually:

    a. a leafy vegetable

    b. peas

    c. pistachio ice cream

10. My grocery cart is more likely to be filled with:

    a. vegetables and fruits

    b. cookies, candy, and ice cream

    c. fat-free cookies, sugar-free candy, and nonfat ice cream

11. How many different foods did you eat yesterday?

    a. over a dozen

    b. one half to one dozen

    c. Does a dozen assorted donuts count as twelve different foods?

12. If the phrase "you are what you eat" was literally true, I would be:

    a. a farmer's market

    b. a Godiva chocolate store

    c. a jar of mayonnaise

You may have smiled at some of the (c) answers, but they are exaggerated truths for many of us, reflecting our fears, obsessions, and extremes with food. Obviously, the greater number of (a) answers you circled, the more variety you have in your diet, and the more your food choices will positively affect your menopausal experience.

As you continue through this chapter, you'll discover why I chose to ask these multiple choice questions. A healthy diet for menopause is not void of fat, sugar, and your favorite foods. It's filled with fruits, vegetables, fluids, some fat, some protein, and a lot of your favorite foods—even if they are loaded with fat.

With chocolate chastised, butter banished, red meat in retreat, and eggs in exile, today's most popular eating rule may be "fat-free," but not for long and certainly not for menopausal women.

DO YOU HAVE A FAT-FREE CHIP ON YOUR SHOULDER?

Almost every woman I've ever met is walking around with a fat-free chip on her shoulder. I have a friend who refuses to join me for pizza because it's too high in fat, a client who panics when her kids bring home potato chips, and another client who canceled her trip to France because she feared the cheese, butter, and cream sauces. Our paralyzing fat phobia has caused us to miss out on the finer things in life—dinners with friends, snacks with our family, and exciting vacations away from home. Our fear of fat has also caused immense guilt and remorse when we do give in and eat some.

Just last week, a guilt-ridden woman called me up with a frantic confession. "I've blown it. I can't believe I did it. I went into the kitchen when everyone was in bed, quietly did my dirty deed, and cleaned up all the evidence so no one would know." It sounds like this woman committed a heinous crime. In her mind she did: She ate real ice cream with huge chunks of chocolate chips.

I get confessions like this all the time from women who tell me that they "were bad yesterday" or they "ate at Burger King last night" or they "secretly ate a Dove bar for lunch." Sometimes I feel like a meal minister: women confess their food sins hoping to be either absolved or punished.

Why do we feel this way about fat, a natural and necessary component of our diet? We have been convinced that eating fat is a vice, that anything void of fat is virtuous, and that if we eat fat we must carry the guilt not only on our shoulders, but also on our hips.

To prevent any wrongdoing and weight gain, many of us turn to the thousands of fat-free, and therefore guilt-free, foods now on the market. We pile our grocery carts high with reduced-fat snacks, nonfat cakes, low-fat cookies, and fat-free dressings, sauces, and spreads. For our canine friends, we even buy reduced-fat dog food. Three-quarters of all Americans (and many of their pets) now consume reduced-fat foods. I'll let you in on a little secret: I'm not one of them. I don't like the taste or consistency of most reduced-fat foods. Food satisfaction is very important to me, and I often find them either too sweet or salty because of the added sugar and sodium. And, I'm sort of doing my own little boycott. I believe that we are designed to eat food that naturally contains some fat. I also know that I'm mentally and physically healthier eating a moderate amount of fat. When I don't get enough, my mood deteriorates until I eat some chips or a piece of chocolate to satisfy my body's need for fat.

It's not easy being a "full-fat" person. It takes longer to grocery shop to make sure that I don't grab the low-fat (except for milk), reduced-fat, or fat-free versions. And I sometimes get looks from other shoppers when they see my cart filled with real food while theirs are filled with the so-called healthier fat-free alternatives. What they don't realize is that most of the fat-free choices are just as high in calories as the regular versions.

Not long ago, I went into a popular bagel store to buy a midmorning snack and was asked if I wanted cream cheese. I replied, "Yes, but I want regular cream cheese, not the lite or low fat." "You do?" they asked in surprise. I actually held up the line while they searched for a container of regular cream cheese buried below all the low-fat varieties. I don't fear fat; I fear that fat will someday become extinct.

There's a follow-up to my bagel experience. As I sat eating my bagel, I noticed that all the low-fat cream cheese eaters had a good-sized inch of it on their bagels. I had taken most of my regular cream cheese off. I also noticed that those who had the most low-fat cream cheese piled on their bagels also carried the most weight on their bodies.

Eating less fat is not the secret to weight loss. Choosing lower-fat foods does not guarantee a lower-fat body. If it did, millions of women would be dropping pounds. Instead, we're adding pounds because we're eating too much of these low-fat foods, or we're eating more food later in the day thinking we have calories to spare. Penn State did the first eye-opening study on the effects of low-fat foods on our eating habits. When yogurt was labeled low fat (whether or not it actually was), women ate significantly more later that day and consumed more total calories. Since then many other studies have shown that when we eat low-fat or nonfat foods, we eat more of them, eat more later, consume more calories, and gain more weight.

As our fat intake has gone down over the last four decades, our weights have increased. Our fat intake has decreased from 41 percent to 34 percent of our total calories—while the incidence of obesity has increased from 25 percent to 33 percent.

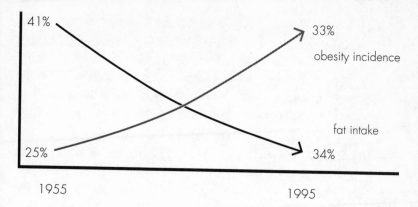

If our fat intake has decreased, shouldn't we be losing weight? First of all, as I've already mentioned, we may be eating less fat, but we're consuming more total calories. The latest food consumption surveys have found that we're eating 200 to 300 more calories than we did ten years ago. Those additional calories may be fat-free, but that doesn't matter. Once excess calories enter our bodies, they are converted to fat and stored as fat. Another explanation for our higher weights is that fat deprivation triggers the starvation response: our metabolism slows down and our fat cells speed up storage to ensure survival.

When I shared this lower fat/higher weight enigma with Cheryl, she did her own personal analysis. "You're right. My friends who eat some fat are leaner than my friends who eat no fat. I was leaner when I allowed myself to eat some fat. Maybe I should reintroduce some fat into my diet to appease my fat cells."

If you've eliminated fat from your diet, I do recommend adding back some fat for both weight loss and general health. As arguments against fat are being chiseled away, there are fewer reasons to eliminate it completely and more reasons to keep some.

- *The New England Journal of Medicine* recently reviewed the results of seven studies totaling 337,819 women and concluded that a low-fat diet (even less than 20 percent of the calories coming from fat) did not lower breast cancer risk. What's more, the vitamin E and essential fatty acids in fat have been found to reduce the risk of breast cancer.

- Not all high-fat diets are linked to heart disease. The Greeks have a high-fat diet, mostly coming from olive oil, and have a lower risk of heart disease. And the French have a high-fat diet, mostly coming from cheese, butter, and cream, and have half the risk we do.

- A very low-fat diet (less than 20 percent of the total calories derived from fat) has been found to reduce estrogen levels and increase menopausal discomfort. Women report more anxiety, irritability, and stress.

- Essential fatty acids are needed to manufacture hormones (including estrogen), build cell membranes, and transmit nerve impulses. They also keep the skin and vaginal tissue healthy. Concerned about wrinkles? Don't cut fat intake too low and include some fat every day.

If fat is so beneficial to midlife women, why all the fuss about fat? Because newspapers, magazines, and television are our primary sources of nutrition information, and fat attracts twice as much coverage as any other nutrition topic. Eating less fat has superseded the more important goal of eating more healthfully. Too much fat isn't healthy, but we've taken it to the extreme and need to realize that too little isn't healthy either, especially during perimenopause. You'll deprive your body of important fat-soluble vitamins, manufacture less estrogen, cause more menopausal tension, trigger a drop in metabolism, and store more fat as your fat cells try to produce additional estrogen. **Your menopausal body can't function well on a staple of fat-free foods.**

Now, it's not just fat-free *foods* we have to worry about, but fat-free *fat*. Olestra (or as it is called on the market, Olean) has been found to decrease the absorption of beta carotene as well as cause diarrhea, intestinal cramping, anal leakage (just typing the words brings up the undesirable image), and what's called fecal urgency. When you've got to go, you really have to go. I'll take some fat over anal leakage and fecal urgency any day.

So take the fat-free chip off your shoulder and let go of any food fears. Fat does not directly cause disease or weight gain unless you overeat it. But, if you consume a moderate amount (a handful!) of chips or other high fat food, they will be quickly utilized by your body before they ever have a chance to damage your arteries or be deposited into your fat cells. While you're at it, take the sugar-free chip off your shoulder, too. Remember: It's not what you eat, but how much you eat that affects the size of your fat cells and your health.

Can you have your fat-free cake and eat it too? Maybe a slice, but not the whole thing. And not if your body is demanding real cake with real fat and sugar and real frosting. The fat-free version will never be as satisfying or substitute for the real thing.

MIND YOUR MENOPAUSAL FOOD CRAVINGS

Every woman knows what it means to have a food craving. We've had them since puberty, we've had them every month premenstrually, and we've had them with any pregnancies. Now that we're in menopause, food cravings are climaxing in intensity and frequency. Are you experiencing the power of menopausal food cravings?

- "I never really liked candy, but now I'm buying jelly beans, licorice, and taffy to make sure I have a ready supply."

- "My body has always seemed to love chocolate, but now it has a head over heels infatuation with it."

- "When I get a craving for my daily bread and butter, I've got to have it! Jam doesn't work; reduced-fat margarine doesn't work. I cannot live by bread alone—I need the butter with it."

- "I feel like I'm pregnant again. I get cravings for pickles, peanuts, and pomegranates just like I did when I was carrying my son for nine months. Where are these cravings coming from?"

Food cravings originate in your hypothalamus, the same structure in your brain that controls reproduction and moods. What we crave is closely tied to what our reproductive system is doing, and what we eat directly influences our moods.

During the ten- to twenty-year transition to menopause, our reproductive systems are winding down with intermittent bursts of overactivity. Sometimes low levels of sex hormones are produced, and other times hormonal levels are skyrocketing. This hormonal roller coaster affects certain brain chemicals in your hypothalamus. These chemicals can make you laugh one minute and cry the next, and they can trigger a need for chocolate one day and chicken the next.

Hundreds of brain chemicals are in a state of flux from your ever-changing hormones, but the three that dramatically affect your menopausal cravings and mood are serotonin, the endorphins, and dopamine. As estrogen and progesterone levels decrease during menopause, so do these mood-enhancing brain chemicals.

- **When serotonin levels are low,** you may feel stressed or depressed, and any carbohydrate, starch, or sugar will increase brain levels. Today, you might crave a bagel and tomorrow bon-bons, but in the end you'll feel uplifted and calm.

- **When endorphin levels are low,** you may feel moody and tired, and any fat, saturated or unsaturated, will increase brain levels. Today, you might desire an avocado and tomorrow some butter on your bread, but the result is that you'll feel energized and euphoric.

- **When dopamine levels are low,** you may have a difficult time concentrating, and any protein, animal or vegetable, will increase brain levels. Today, you might yearn for tenderloin; tomorrow tofu (some women do), and you'll be rewarded with more brain power.

Food cravings are the *only* way for your brain to communicate exactly what it needs to function most optimally. Food cravings are a blessing, not a curse. I realize that when we are gaining unwanted weight, our first thought is to restrict our food intake and fight our food cravings. Let that thought pass. Restriction will only cause more weight gain because food cravings can't be quelled; they only intensify, and you'll end up eating more sugar, starch, or fat when you can't take it any longer. Instead, recognize the benefits of your cravings and satisfy them immediately with a small amount. **Carbohydrates, fat, and protein are your "feel good" foods that boost your "feel good" brain chemicals.**

Of all the brain chemicals, serotonin may be the most influential for menopausal women. Low levels have been linked to many of the menopausal complaints: sleep difficulties, depression, mood swings, memory loss, headaches, increased premenstrual tension, and even hot flashes. By listening to your food cravings and using carbohydrates to boost serotonin, you'll experience a noticeable difference in how you feel. If you ignore your carbohydrate cravings, serotonin will drop even more and so will your energy level, moods, and memory. For more information on the intriguing connection between brain chemicals, cravings, and mood, you may wish to consult another of my books, *Why Women Need Chocolate*.

Speaking of chocolate, it's the number one food craved by menopausal women. What is it about chocolate? Chocolate has the perfect combination of sugar and fat to increase both serotonin and the endorphins simultaneously. Another chemical in chocolate, phenylethylamine, stimulates the pleasure centers in our brain and mimics the feeling of falling in love. Simply put: **Chocolate is your menopausal mood stabilizer.**

What about the negative effects of chocolate? Like any other food, unless you overeat it, are allergic to it, or get migraines from it (or don't brush your teeth after eating it), there are no negative effects. Chocolate does not cause acne, nor does it clog our arteries. A recent discovery is that chocolate contains antioxidents, which help to decrease heart disease risk by keeping our arteries clean. In the larger picture of eating a variety of foods and exercising—there's always room for chocolate.

But there's more to menopausal food cravings than chocolate and brain chemicals. A few years ago, I conducted a food craving survey on over five hundred premenopausal and menopausal women. You'll be pleased to hear that it's not just chocolate, carbohydrates, protein, and fat we crave during the transition. We also crave more vegetables and fruits. In fact, menopausal women were 30 percent more likely to crave vegetables and 27 percent more likely to crave fruit. Our midlife bodies crave foods that will enhance our well-being, and fruits and vegetables not only contain vital nutrients, they also contain natural sources of estrogen.

EAT YOUR ESTROGEN

Just a few years ago, I never would have thought I would be able to advise women to "eat" their estrogen. But the science of nutrition is relatively new, and a recent entry is here to stay: phytoestrogens. You may have read about them in magazine articles or books, but what exactly are they and where do you find them? *Phyto* means plant, and over three hundred plants have thus far been found to contain weak estrogens that have 1/100 to 1/1000 the strength of the estrogen your body produces. They are too weak to compensate fully for the drop of estrogen during menopause, but when eaten daily in sufficient amounts, they are strong enough to provide the following benefits to your physical and psychological health:

- Researchers at Bowman Gray School of Medicine have discovered that phytoestrogens reduce the severity of hot flashes. Other studies have found that they decrease menopausal anxiety, irritability, and mood swings.

- The University of Kentucky found that plant estrogens reduced the LDL (bad) cholesterol by 13 percent and overall heart disease risk by 18 percent.

- The University of Illinois found that phytoestrogens increased bone density by 3 percent.

- Studies on Japanese women reveal that they have a 400 percent lower risk of breast cancer than we do, and the primary reason may be their high intake of phytoestrogens. Japanese women also have an easier transition. Their most common menopausal complaints are graying hair and stiff shoulders, and they don't even have a word for "hot flash."

- Studies on fat cell metabolism have found that the more phytoestrogens we eat, the less work our fat cells have to do. Japanese women only gain an average of four pounds during the transition while we gain twelve pounds. *Phytoestrogens fight fat cells.*

So what can you eat to get these famous phytoestrogens? Most women are turning specifically to soy products because Japanese women eat them in quantity, and they are the healthiest women in the world, with the greatest longevity and the lowest rates of breast cancer, heart disease, and osteoporosis. Your first encounter with soy products may be tentative, and you may have to do some experimentation with cooking. To help, I have included some recent cookbooks in the Suggested Reading section.

(Nina Shandler's *Estrogen the Natural Way* is filled with innovative and tasty recipes.) But new products are hitting the marketplace all the time, and new ways to use soybeans are being introduced to this country. We can call it the "Soy of Cooking," and here are a few ideas to get you started:

- You can go the more traditional route with tofu, stir-frying it with vegetables and adding it to soups.
- You can add silken tofu to salad dressings, cream soups, sauces, and casseroles.
- You can use tofu of any kind to fill Mexican dishes such as tacos and burritos or to stuff Italian dishes such as ravioli and cannelloni.
- You can bake anything with soy flour, replacing one-quarter of the regular flour called for.
- You can go the convenient route:
  - drink soy milk or eat soy cheese and yogurt
  - use soybean oil in cooking
  - marinate and add flavor with soy sauce and teriyaki sauce
  - buy soy deli meats and burgers
  - buy roasted soy nuts for an afternoon snack
  - sprinkle soy protein on cereals or add it to beverages (It's tasteless.)
  - go to Japanese restaurants and order miso soup, tempe, and other dishes
- Or, you can experiment with some of the high-tech products such as soy pizza, soy grits, soy ice cream, and Beanut butter (this is not a typo), which is a nut spread made from soybeans.

From milk to nuts—soybeans are extremely versatile. Many of these products can be found in grocery stores, and even more choice can be found in Asian food stores, health food stores, and natural food supermarkets.

How much should you eat? The general recommendation is to consume between 30 and 100 mg of phytoestrogens a day. You'll be hard pressed to find the phytoestrogen content on nutrition labels or in most nutrition books. If you rely on soy products, three ounces of tofu, two tablespoons of soy protein powder, or one glass of soy milk a day will meet the minimal recommendation.

If tofu is intolerable to your taste buds or can only be tolerated a couple of times a week, flaxseeds also have a high phytoestrogen content. They have a nutty flavor and can be used in baking or ground and sprinkled on just about anything. Another way to make sure that you're getting your plant estrogens is to simply eat plants. The USDA started recommending five servings of fruits and vegetables a day long before phytoestrogens were even discovered. And phytoestrogens are just one group of hundreds of other beneficial chemicals found in plants. Called *phytochemicals*, these substances are not quite vitamins and not quite minerals, but they are nutrients that our bodies need to maximize health. I could go through an extensive list of fruits and vegetables, outlining which contain what phytochemicals, but the lycopene, lutein, terpenes, indoles, flavonoids, and quercetin (to mention just a few of the strange sounding names) all do about the same thing in our bodies—make us healthy. They reduce disease risk by cleaning our arteries, lowering blood pressure, boosting our immune systems, and slowing down the aging process.

Eat as many fruits and vegetables as possible and aim for at least five servings a day. Don't feel too overwhelmed, a serving is much smaller than you think: usually four ounces of juice, a half cup of vegetables, and a medium-size fruit. If you drink an eight-ounce glass of juice for breakfast, include a fruit at lunch, and eat a cup of broccoli at dinner—that's five servings!

Only 20 percent of women age 35 to 54 are getting the five a day they need. If you're one of the 80 percent who aren't, the following suggestions will help you ease produce into your daily cuisine:

- Squeeze one-half a lemon or orange into your glass of water.
- Make it a habit to top your cereal with fruit.
- Start your day with juice (at least a quick glass before your coffee).
- Snack on fruit: blueberries, strawberries, plums, oranges, papaya, and grapes have the highest phytochemical content.
- Frequent the juice bars and smoothie establishments.
- Have fruit pie for dessert, fruit tarts, apple strudel, fruit sorbets, or chocolate-covered strawberries.
- Order vegetables on your pizza.
- Keep a ready supply of frozen vegetables in your freezer for those days you can't make it to the market. (Frozen vegetables have the same phytochemical and nutrient content as fresh.)
- Turn over a new leaf: instead of iceberg lettuce, use spinach, bok choy, kale, collard greens, arugula, escarole, radicchio, mustard greens, Swiss chard, and broccoli. The darker the leaf, the more phytochemicals and nutrients.

What if these new leaves taste bitter? What if you were born to hate broccoli? The University of Michigan had women taste-test a variety of the more bitter dark green, leafy vegetables and found that about 25 percent could barely get beyond the first bite, 25 percent barely noticed the bitter flavor, and the rest fell in between. To make these greens more pleasing to your palate, cooking them in a small amount of oil or adding vinegar will help take off their bitter edge.

I've had a number of clients who were concerned about the pesticide residues on produce, so you may be too. The consensus is that you're better off eating fruits and vegetables with pesticides than eating no fruits and vegetables. But to be on the safe side, buy organic when you can. And when you can't, wash them with water and mild dishwashing detergent and rinse well. Soap residue isn't healthy either.

If you need more encouragement to eat fruits and vegetables and get your five a day, they also contain fiber, vitamin C, beta carotene, zinc, boron, magnesium, and folic acid—all important nutrients for your menopausal body. In addition, they are loaded with water, and water may be the most vital nutrient for your changing body.

WET YOUR APPETITE

Next to oxygen, water is the most necessary substance for life. You can live without soy products, you can live without fruits and vegetables (although not very well), and you can even live without chocolate—or at least some people can—but you can't live without water.

Water is your coolant, lubricant, solvent, and transportation system. It regulates body temperature, maintains body fluids, carries nutrients, removes waste, and is the medium for every cellular reaction. Over half of your body is made up of water: 80 percent of your blood is water, 75 percent of your brain is water, and 70 percent of your muscle mass is water. When you get dehydrated, the negative result affects your ability to think, exercise, sleep, work, and play. Dehydration also affects your risk of disease because your blood volume is decreased and the concentration of cholesterol, fats, glucose, and waste products increases.

Children, the elderly, burn victims, pregnant women, and menopausal women are most prone to dehydration. During the transition, hot flashes and muscle breakdown cause additional water loss, and such effects of dehydration as heart palpitations, dizziness, headaches, constipation, dry skin, and lethargy become more severe. In fact, dehydration is a common cause of midlife fatigue. And the remedy may be as simple as sipping water.

How much should you sip? Enough to make your urine pale in color. The widely accepted eight-glass-a-day recommendation has little scientific basis. Depending on body size and metabolism, some women are still dehydrated after eight glasses; others are adequately hydrated with five glasses. If you're not drinking enough water, your urine becomes dark in color and low in volume, putting a strain on your kidneys and increasing the likelihood of urinary tract infections, in addition to the other negative effects of dehydration.

Drinking adequate fluids can also help you outsmart your menopausal fat cells. Because hunger is often confused with thirst, we end up eating when we really need to be drinking and storing fat in our fat cells when our other cells really needed to be hydrated with water. By sipping water throughout the day, you'll be assured that hunger is a message to eat and that what you eat will be burned instead of stored.

Sipping water may sound simple, but any new habit takes a while to adopt. Here are some ways to wet your appetite and hydrate your menopausal body:

- Eat produce—the five-a-day recommendation is equivalent to at least one glass of water.

- Keep a bottle of water with you or a glass of water nearby at all times.

- If your office doesn't already have a water cooler, lobby to get one and get one for your home as well.

- If you find water bland, squeeze in some lemon or lime juice, throw in an orange slice, or add some sugar. A little sugar can help with absorption.

- If you are concerned about chlorine, parasites, or any other substance potentially found in water supplies, your best bet is to get a water filter. There's no guarantee that bottled water is free of contaminants.

- Drink other fluids: juices, electrolyte drinks, milk, flavored water, and lemonade. These take a little longer to be absorbed, so water is still the best.

- Don't count coffee, tea, iced tea, and alcohol as hydrating liquids. Caffeine and alcohol are both diuretics that rob your body of water.

Coffee and alcohol don't count as hydrating liquids, but can you drink them? Aren't they unhealthy for menopausal women?

Let's talk about caffeine first. After decades of research, most of the news on coffee is good to the last drop. A Harvard study on 85,000 women followed for ten years found no association between caffeine, blood cholesterol, and heart disease. Unfiltered coffee does increase blood cholesterol, but as long as you use a filter to capture the oils, you're safe even at six cups a day. In addition, little, if any, conclusive evidence exists linking caffeine to benign breast lumps, kidney stones, hot flashes, and even osteoporosis. Caffeine has little impact on fracture rates as long as you're getting enough calcium. Caffeine binds calcium and causes it to be excreted in your urine, but one cup of coffee causes only a 5 mg calcium loss.

Not only does caffeine not produce the risks once thought, it may actually be beneficial to your moods and well-being. Caffeine has been found to alleviate migraines and improve concentration, short-term memory, and depression. A highly publicized Harvard study discovered that those women who drank two to three cups of coffee a day were 70 percent less likely to commit suicide compared to those who didn't drink any. No correlation was found in men.

Even though the research says caffeine is okay, your body may not. Caffeine is a stimulant, and some women feel that it triggers their hot flashes, increases breast tenderness, and/or interferes with sleep. Because some women are more sensitive to caffeine than others, I suggest trying an experiment: Give up coffee for a month and see how you feel. The first week or so you may experience withdrawal, but after that you may discover that you feel better when your body is caffeine-free.

So with coffee, there appears to be no grounds for concern as long as you use a filter, consume enough calcium (more on calcium in the next section), and are not oversensitive to caffeine.

Now, what about alcohol? With alcohol, too, we raise our glasses to toast the benefits. They include:

- **Lower rates of heart disease.** Up to two drinks per day increase HDLs and cut heart disease risk in half.

- **Stable weight.** Up to two drinks a day have no effect on weight or body fat, unless you are the type of person who eats more when you consume alcohol.

- **Lower death rates.** As few as one to three drinks a week reduce the likelihood of early death by 17 percent.

Needless to say, moderation is the key. One to three drinks a week is all you need to get the benefits that stem from the phytochemicals found in alcohol. More than two drinks a day, and the risks to your liver, breasts, and longevity escalate and outweigh the benefits. The effects of alcohol on health are best described as a J-shaped curve. Those who don't drink at all have slightly higher death rates; those who drink moderately have reduced rates, but those who drink in excess have much higher death rates. The Nurses' Health Study found that heavy drinkers (more than fourteen drinks a week) had a 20 percent higher death rate.

Heavy drinking is worse for women because we have less of the enzyme, alcohol dehydrogenase, that detoxifies the alcohol. This is especially true during the premenstrual time and the menopausal transition. As estrogen levels drop during midlife, so does the activity of this enzyme. When 20- and 60-year-old women consume the same amount of alcohol, the 60-year-old women will have a 20 percent higher blood alcohol level. This may explain why excessive alcohol consumption is more strongly linked to breast cancer and liver disease as we grow older.

How can you get the benefit to your heart without harming your breasts or liver? Through moderation: One to three drinks a week will give you all the benefits without the risks. One drink is 5 ounces of wine, 12 ounces of beer, or 1½ ounces of hard liquor. We used to think that red wine was the only winner. The latest research suggests that white wine, beer, and hard liquor also provide similar benefits. This finding doesn't mean that if you don't drink, you should start having cocktails every night and wine with your dinner. Alcohol can disrupt sleep patterns and trigger headaches, and other lifestyle habits are far more important to adopt than taking up drinking. Studies are finding that red grape juice and nonalcoholic wines still have some of the beneficial phytochemicals without the potentially harmful alcohol.

Right now, you're probably thinking, "Wait a minute! Every book and article I've ever read recommends avoidance of caffeine, alcohol, fat, sugar, and chocolate for a healthier menopause. Now you're telling me that not only can I enjoy these things again, they may actually be beneficial!?"

The truth is that many health professionals rely on the old standby recommendations for healthy eating: no caffeine, alcohol, fat, sugar, and sodium. But the old standbys are just that—old. I have shared with you the latest information on how foods and beverages affect your changing body. Elimination isn't the goal; enlightenment is. Lori's enlightenment came after realizing that the more she restricted her diet, the more out-of-sorts she felt and the more weight she gained.

EAT WELL FOR "A CHANGE"

So far, we've discussed the importance of eating some fat, responding to your food cravings, getting your daily dose of phytoestrogens and other phytochemicals, drinking plenty of water, and consuming a moderate amount of coffee and alcohol. There are two other food areas that are important to midlife women: protein and calcium.

Protein is a Greek word meaning primary or holding first place, which stresses its importance in our diets. Every cell needs protein. Every enzyme is made up of protein, and your immune system relies on protein to stay strong. For these functions, your body needs a minimum of 25 to 30 grams of protein a day. One cheeseburger provides over 30 grams: 23 for the patty, 7 for the cheese, and 2.5 in the bun. The Recommended Dietary Allowances doubles the minimum need to 50 to 60 grams as a safeguard. As a menopausal woman, you need that extra protein to recharge your immune system and rebuild your muscle with your strength training program.

To get your 60 grams of protein a day, include two servings a day from a variety of different sources. What type of protein should you eat?

- Red meat? Something about it seems to be associated with cancer and heart disease, but after thirty years of research, we still don't know if it's the saturated fat or something else in red meat. A couple of servings a week will not produce any detrimental effects. Unless, of course, it's ground beef that has been contaminated with *E. coli* and isn't cooked to well-done. The recent outbreaks have made all of us cautious about the meats and other foods we choose.

- Fish? There's something fishy going on with fish. We used to worry about the high fat content of salmon, trout, and other fish, but we now know that the omega-3 fatty acids in fish oil are beneficial to our health and can help with heart disease, some cancers, and vaginal dryness.

- Shellfish? We can eat shrimp, clams, oysters, and lobster again. Their high cholesterol content does not become cholesterol in our blood unless we add a lot of fat to them with butter and sauces.

- Fowl? Chicken and turkey have a slightly higher protein content than beef, and therefore, are a great way to get your protein.

- Pork? It's being called the other white meat, reducing blood cholesterol as much, if not more, than poultry.

- Eggs? According to the American Heart Association, you can now eat four a week.

- Vegetable sources? Legumes and grains are not complete proteins (soybeans come the closest), so if you've switched to a strict vegetarian diet, you need to make sure that you combine your beans and rice. Consult a dietitian, your physician, or a vegetarian cookbook on how best to combine your protein sources.

You can eat a variety of vegetable and animal proteins to benefit your midlife body, but don't confuse adequate protein with high protein. Too much protein may leach calcium from your body and cause bone loss. When 86,000 women were studied, those who ate about 100 grams of protein a day had a 22 percent higher fracture rate than those who ate 60 grams a day. Yet another reason for midlife women to think twice before considering a very high-protein diet. It could increase our risk for osteoporosis.

Which brings me to your other important midlife need: calcium. Women start to lose calcium from their bones at age 30. We lose about 1 percent each year until we stop menstruating, then we lose 2 to 3 percent each year for the next ten years. Because of this accelerated bone loss, your need for calcium increases from 1,000 mg a day during the transition to 1,200 to 1,500 mg after. And calcium is not just for your bones. It's also a natural relaxer, may help with sleep, and may reduce the risk of colon cancer. For all these reasons, make a commitment to consuming adequate calcium.

Milk products have the highest calcium content and therefore, are often the easiest way to get your 1,000 to 1,500 mg a day. But if you are allergic to milk, don't like it, or hold the belief that milk is more of a menace than a must, there are many other ways to get your calcium.

1 cup milk	300 mg
1 cup cornmeal	483 mg
8 oz. calcium-fortified orange juice	300 mg
1/2 cup tofu	250 mg
1/2 cup dry-roasted soybeans	232 mg
3 tablespoons flaxseed	76 mg
1 cup dried figs	287 mg
1 cup bok choy	165 mg
8 oz. mineral water	100 mg
2 corn tortillas	88 mg
1 cup broccoli	80 mg
1 milk chocolate bar	80 mg

To get your 1,500 mg of calcium a day, you'd have to drink 5 glasses of milk or 15 glasses of mineral water (actually, drinking mineral water is an easy way to add calcium). You'd have to eat 27 ounces of tofu, 19 cups of broccoli, or 19 milk chocolate bars. Other than the chocolate, these amounts are unappealing and impossible. So we start counting on calcium supplements to save our bones.

Can you rely on calcium supplements? Some, but not entirely. Foods contain all the necessary ingredients for adequate absorption, and studies have shown that food sources of calcium increase bone density at a 50 percent higher rate than supplements. If you do take supplements, calcium carbonate and calcium citrate are most recommended. Calcium citrate is better absorbed, but you have to take more pills. Calcium carbonate has to be taken with meals to increase absorption.

What about supplements in general? We popped 10 billion of them last year, and the vitamin aisle is overwhelming. Just by its sheer size, we should be the best-nourished people in the world. But we're not because vitamin supplements lack nutrients. Phytochemicals and phytoestrogens were just recently discovered, and most supplements do not contain them. My bet is that hundreds of other nutrients haven't been discovered yet, and supplements will never replace the benefits of eating.

If you take supplements, use them to give added insurance, not to replace food. And when choosing supplements:

- **Ignore the hype.** There is nothing natural about any pill and little difference in how they are absorbed or utilized by the body.

- **Ignore the claims.** They do not miraculously cure disease, prevent aging, or reduce stress. And the vitamins "formulated specifically for menopause" do not miraculously "alleviate the symptoms." Vitamin E and the B vitamins do have some evidence supporting the claim that they help with hot flashes and mood changes, but other studies have shown little benefit.

- **Ignore the arguments.** The most common one is that our soil is depleted of nutrients, so we must take supplements. If the soil is truly depleted, the plants wouldn't grow anyway. Fertilizers mineralize the soil, so in those areas where soil has a lower mineral content, fertilizers more than compensate.

- ***Don't* ignore food.** All studies have shown that fruits and vegetables decrease disease risk, but supplement studies have failed to hold up. After reviewing over two hundred studies, researchers found that those who ate the most fruits and vegetables had one-half the risk of developing cancer than those who ate the least.

Get your nutrients the old-fashioned way—eat them! While you're eating and making meno-positive food choices, keep one important principle in mind: **Eat a wide variety of foods,** including those that are high in protein and calcium, those that you crave, and especially those that are in the fruit and vegetable family. Plants provide phytoestrogens and phytochemicals, are naturally high in every nutrient your changing body needs, are loaded with water and fiber, and are naturally low in calories and fat, helping you to moderate your fat intake. Whew! The benefits of produce are endless!

Variety has always been the basis of healthy eating. As Virginia Woolf wrote in 1929, "One cannot think well, sleep well, or love well if one has not dined well." Now during menopause, you have even more reason to heed that advice and eat well for "a change." Every food will help you to accomplish this goal, whether it's chocolate, cheese, Chinese food, carrots, or cantaloupe. The next time you get hungry, check in with your body to see if it's requesting any particular food. If it is, then give yourself permission to eat the food and experience the benefits to your body and brain.

HOW WILL YOU MAXIMIZE MENO-POSITIVE FOOD CHOICES?

Unlike most books, the emphasis of this chapter was not on reducing fat, red meat, sugar, sodium, caffeine, and alcohol. It was on using food to balance your body and brain and enhance your well-being. Remember: There are no good or bad food choices—just conscious decisions about how you nourish your midlife body.

Check all of the following food choice options that you want to commit to, and you'll be on your way to eating well for "a change":

❏ I will consider fat a healthy component of my diet.

❏ I will think of my favorite foods as healthy food choices.

❏ I will eat only the fat-free foods that are satisfying to me.

❏ Regardless of the fat content, I will eat no more than a handful of the foods that I choose.

❏ I will check in with my body and identify whether or not I am craving any particular food.

❏ I will trust my body's need for chocolate, fat, protein, and sugar.

❏ I will be more aware of my body's cravings for vegetables and fruits.

❏ I will not categorize foods as "good" or "bad" and will consider all food choices healthy food choices.

❏ I will focus on eating plant sources of estrogen.

❏ I will experiment with soy products.

❏ I will commit to eating five servings of fruits and vegetables a day.

❏ I will adequately hydrate my body by sipping water throughout the day.

❏ I will consume caffeine and alcohol in moderation.

❏ I will eat two quality protein sources every day.

❑ I will focus on food sources of calcium and take supplements only as necessary to reach 1,500 mg a day.

❑ I will get my nutrients the old-fashioned way—by eating them.

❑ I will take the next step of living a meno-positive lifestyle by reading the next chapter.

chapter eight

LIVING A
MENO-POSITIVE LIFESTYLE

The word lifestyle is all encompassing—it's your personal style of going through life: your priorities, behaviors, method of operating, and philosophy of living. Everything you've accomplished so far with The Meno-Positive Approach, from your newly acquired attitudes to your enhanced eating and exercise habits, means that you have a more positive method of going through one of life's most important transitions: menopause. You are making choices that will realistically manage midlife weight gain, smooth your menopausal transition, and render a general sense of well-being.

But you can do even more. Living a meno-positive lifestyle means taking care of your body and mind in the best possible way. This chapter will offer a variety of additional ways to further strengthen your physical and emotional well-being—including options to balance your life, stay connected to your needs, recharge your battery, calm your mind, relax your muscles, add happiness and laughter, and, perhaps most important, reduce stress.

Every woman I know wants to have more balance, energy, and happiness, but the number one factor that prevents us from accomplishing these positive goals is *stress*. It zaps our energy so that we're too exhausted to exercise. It robs us of time so that we can't relax and enjoy the things we're doing. It forces us to rely on quick fixes like caffeine, alcohol, sugar, and fast food so that we can make it through the struggles of the day. It causes us to lose sleep, lose our tempers, lose our perspective, and generally lose our health. When stress is ongoing and relentless, it wreaks havoc with our bodies by overstimulating our hearts, weakening our immune systems, and upsetting our hormonal balance. Because stress diminishes estrogen levels, it has been linked to menstrual dysfunction, infertility, intense PMS, megamenopause, and excess weight gain. As you know from chapter 2, our fat cells respond to stress by growing bigger, stronger, and more resilient as they try to compensate with more estrogen production. Therefore, **outwitting stress is an effective way to outsmart your fat cells.**

Do you feel stressed right now? Probably an unnecessary question for most of us because stress occupies the majority of our waking hours and often interferes with our sleeping hours. The average person encounters fifty stressful situations a day, the first occurring when the alarm startles us out of slumber and the last when we're anxiously trying to fall asleep. Simply taking the time to read this book may be producing stress because you're worried about the clothes that need to be washed, the shopping that needs to be done, the argument that needs to be resolved, the bills that need to be paid, the paperwork that needs to be completed, and the deadlines that need to be met. Many of us put in more than eight hours a day at work, then come home to start our second shift with an endless list of family and home responsibilities.

No wonder we have difficulty finding the time to get a haircut; take a bath; get together with friends; spend quality time with our families; get to the gynecologist for our annual exams; go for a walk; lift weights; eat small, frequent meals; or even relax on the couch. The frenetic American lifestyle gets in the way.

On top of the time-consuming, anxiety-producing work and family-related stressors, midlife women have a huge additional stress: *menopause*. During the ten- to twenty-year transition, every single cell in your body is trying to adjust to lower estrogen levels, and this internal turmoil makes you physiologically stressed. Stress can come from external factors (such as taxes and teenagers) or internal factors (such as injury and changing hormones), and we have both kinds of stress interfering with our quality of life. We are biologically upset from diminishing estrogen levels; we are emotionally strained from the weight gain, more visible signs of aging, sleep difficulties, and fatigue; and many of us are traumatically affected by other life-changing events such as divorce, relocation, layoffs, children going off to college, ill parents, or the death of loved ones. The biological changes of menopause interact with the other social changes going on in our lives, making us feel more stressed out than ever before.

Unfortunately, as more and more stress is added to our lives, our bodies become less and less able to cope with it. Researchers at the University of Pittsburgh have found that as estrogen levels decrease, the stress hormone adrenaline increases. Almost everyone gets nervous giving a speech, but when menopausal women were asked to talk in front of a group, their stress hormones, blood pressures, and heart rates rose significantly higher than the premenopausal women. Perhaps our bodies are trying to tell us something: Menopause and stress are not a good mix. The harried, tense, on-the-go lifestyle isn't healthy or worth it any longer. It's time to slow down and welcome tranquillity, relaxation, and balance to our lives.

For a healthier, smoother, and trimmer transition to menopause, let's all think *"less stress."*

LIVE TODAY LESS STRESSED

"To be less stressed, I'd need a house that cleans itself, a live-in assistant, a car that never breaks down, a boss who never has unrealistic expectations, kids who never complain, and a husband who always pitches in to help. I don't have time to practice stress management techniques. I'm too stressed to reduce stress."

This was Rita's initial reaction when we started discussing how she needed to reduce the stress in her life in order to ease her menopausal transition and lose weight. Then she realized that feeling "too stressed to reduce stress" was a warning flag that she better do something—quick.

You may be familiar with the many techniques recommended to help us cope with stress. Having a hobby, playing the piano, listening to music or relaxation tapes, leisure reading, keeping a stress journal, getting a pet, gardening, and, of course, exercising are among them. But coping with menopausal stress requires immediate attention. As Rita said, "These coping skills are all well and good, but I need something that I can do anytime and anywhere. When my menopausal stress hits, I can't wait until my six o'clock karate class. I need to de-stress right then and there or I'll detonate."

Often the best way to learn how to de-stress quickly is through other women's successful experiences, so I polled midlife women on their most effective menopausal stress busters. "Peace and quiet" was the overriding favored method. Here are a few of their unique responses.

Do Not Disturb: I'm Having a Menopausal Moment

Wouldn't it be great if we could put up a Do Not Disturb sign when we're feeling overwhelmed? One woman did just that. Whenever, as she called it, a "menopausal moment" hit, where she lost her cool and perspective, she would hang this sign on her office or bedroom door. Her family and coworkers joked about it, but it was no joke to her. She said that "even a few minutes of peaceful solitude maintains my sanity."

Having time to reflect, regroup, reassess—or just do nothing—is important to all of us, but it's vital during menopause. When we don't have our quiet time, menopausal stress can take over, and life becomes one emergency after another. If you don't feel comfortable putting up a sign, then how about turning off the ringer on your phone for a while, going into the bathroom for some privacy, or sitting in your car for a few minutes? Look for the subliminal message in meno*pause*, and give yourself permission to *pause* every day of your transition.

Ear Plugs and Volume Control

Caroline works in an open office lined with cubicles and lives in a house filled with three teenagers. "I can't stay focused and get work done with everyone talking on the phones, and I can't relax with my kids playing music, watching television, and arguing with each other. Distracting noise is my major stressor. Since I can't turn down the volume of what's going on around me, I literally plug my ears and turn down my stress."

In lieu of putting in earplugs, you could put on earphones and listen to a classical tape or other relaxing music. Because women are more sensitive to noise than men—and we become even more sensitive during the midlife transition—any way we can reduce distracting sounds will help to silence the stress response.

Take a Mini Mind Vacation

When Chrisi can't hop on a plane to a peaceful destination, she imagines one. "Whenever I feel stressed, I close my eyes and envision myself on vacation somewhere relaxing and exotic. Sometimes I'm alone, sometimes I'm with my husband, and sometimes I'm with Mel Gibson—but I'm always on a sandy beach watching the sun set over the ocean."

Visualization can be a powerful tool. Instead of daydreaming about Costa Rica or the Caribbean (with or without a handsome celebrity), some women imagine a bird flying gracefully in the sky, a balloon drifting slowly in the air, or a stream cascading gently over rocks (just typing these pleasant phrases is reducing stress for me). What you imagine doesn't really matter; what matters is that you take yourself out of your stressful surroundings to a place that calms and composes you.

Is This Going to Matter a Year from Now?

I thank one of my clients, Mary Jane, who shared this simple, yet effective technique. I've started using it, so I know it works. When you start obsessing about something and can't let it go (which you are more likely to do during PMS and menopause), ask yourself, "Is this going to matter a year from now?" Is this deadline going to matter? This presentation? This unmade bed? This dirty floor? This dent in my car? This new gray hair I found? This chocolate chip cookie I ate? Ninety-nine percent of the time the answer will be no, and you'll gain perspective and realize what a waste of precious energy and time the situation is causing. If it's something that eventually has to be done, can't it wait a week? A day? An hour? You'll be more productive later if you give yourself time now to go to the gym, go to the movies, or go to the masseuse.

M and Ms—Massage, Muscle Relaxation, Meditation, and Mind Control

For some women, M&Ms mean those wonderful little colorful chocolate-filled candies that they eat when they're under stress, but for Joyce, M and Ms mean practicing mind/body techniques such as meditation, muscle relaxation, and massage.

These centuries-old techniques may be your most effective means of achieving a less stressed lifestyle. With the out-of-control, life-is-passing-me-by way we feel, millions are turning to spas, well-being centers, and meditation retreats, eager to take the journey to heal ourselves, balance our lives, and live each day to its fullest.

MINDFUL MENOPAUSE: NEW AGE MEDICINE FOR MIDDLE AGE

New Age books have flooded the market, mind-body seminars are attracting *Fortune* 500 executives, and "mindfulness" is a rapidly growing buzzword. Even though I haven't called The Meno-Positive Approach "mindful," it definitely fits into the definition of "purposeful attention." Being aware of how your body feels while exercising, staying in tune with your hunger and fullness signals, listening to your body's food messages, and enjoying the eating experience without feeling guilty are all mind-body techniques that increase your internal awareness and keep you anchored to what you are doing.

"Living in the moment" is a popular phrase among mind-body educators, and it's more than New Age mumbo jumbo. Many of us are racing through life without really experiencing it and transitioning through menopause without really learning and growing from it. Instead of obsessing about what happened yesterday or stressing out about what might happen tomorrow, we need to get fulfillment from what's happening right this very instant—whether we're working, playing, eating, exercising, or relaxing. As Joan Borysenko so accurately stated in her revolutionary book, *Minding the Body, Mending the Mind*, "The joy is not in finishing the activity—the joy is in doing it."

The value of using mind-body techniques to slow down and stay connected is quickly gaining recognition among consumers and gaining acceptance within the medical community. Herbert Benson of Harvard Medical School has proven many times over that relaxing the mind triggers a relaxed state in the body. He and his colleagues were the first to document a phenomenon they called "the relaxation response," where heart rate, blood pressure, muscle tension, and oxygen consumption could all be decreased to *below* resting levels. (His books *The Relaxation Response* and *Beyond The Relaxation Response* as well as other books in the Suggested Reading provide a more in-depth explanation.) In addition to Benson's research, many other studies have shown that massage, meditation, deep breathing, and other relaxation skills can counteract the negative effects of stress, decrease PMS severity by up to 58 percent, and reduce hot flashes by as much as 70 percent!

But even with these impressive results, it's important to keep in mind that mind-body techniques are not a cure-all for menopause or any other condition. They are alternative approaches to be used alongside more traditional medical treatments. They are worthwhile options that can help us reduce stress, bring about a restful state, and achieve heightened mental and physical health.

Massage

Hippocrates once said, "The physician must be acquainted with many things, most assuredly rubbing." After thousands of years, we now know why "the father of medicine" considered massage such an integral part of health. It has been found to relieve anxiety and depression, increase breathing in asthmatic people, decrease crying in infants, increase immune function in AIDS patients, and increase serenity in menopausal women. Even those with eating disorders report decreased anxiety and improved body image with weekly massages.

Massage offers these medical benefits because touch is a primal need, as necessary as food, water, clothing, and shelter. We have 5 million touch receptors on our skin that send pleasing messages to our brains. Even one friendly touch on the arm can significantly reduce blood pressure and heart rate.

But Americans don't touch with hugs, gestures, or massage as often as we could. Various countries have been studied for their "touch quotient," and the United States is toward the bottom of the list for touch and near the top of the list for stress, obesity, and chronic diseases. The French touch three times more frequently than we do, using touch as a form of greeting, communication, and public display of affection. They are among the least stressed, most fit people in the world.

Meditation

For many women, just hearing the word *meditation* is intimidating. They think that they have to light incense, stare at a Buddha statue, sit in an uncomfortable yoga position, and chant for an hour. That's the seventies version of meditation. Today, all you need is fifteen minutes and:

1. **A quiet place.** Anywhere will do, including your car, the bathroom, or under a tree.

2. **A comfortable position.** Sit up straight, lie back in a chair, or lie down on the couch, in bed, or in the bathtub.

3. **Rhythmic concentration.** Either focus on your breathing or repeat a word.

Many repeat the word *one*, but any word will do; others repeat the phrase "I am calm" over and over until their minds have no choice but to start believing it. Whatever word or phrase you use, within minutes you'll trigger the relaxation response, increase blood flow to the brain, and feel yourself drifting off to a place that's free of anxiety, stress, and menopause—at least temporarily.

Deep Breathing

You already know how to breathe, it's automatic. But do you know how to deep breathe? When you concentrate on your breathing and purposefully control the timing and depth, it's a form of meditation. Here's how: Breathe deeply from your abdomen (not your chest), watch (or feel with your hand) your abdomen expand when you breathe in through your nose and contract when you breathe out through your mouth. During that exhale, imagine yourself emptying your body of stress and tension, literally breathing a sigh of relief. Even after as few as ten deep breaths, you'll feel noticeably calmer. And when done on a regular basis, deep breathing has been found to reduce hot flashes by 50 percent!

Light Therapy

I had a client who thought light therapy was the opposite of heavy-duty psychotherapy. I was amused by her mistaken definition, but she and many others are not aware of the rejuvenating effects of sunlight. Stepping outside in the sun for as few as fifteen minutes (with sunscreen!) will release the calming brain chemical serotonin and reduce anxiety and stress. All of us can benefit from daily exposure to natural sunlight, and many can greatly benefit from the more clinical use of light therapy. Some promising research has been conducted on the use of specially designed light boxes for the treatment of intense menopause and PMS, seasonal affective disorder, and depression. These light boxes emit rays similar to the sun's, come in various shapes and sizes, and are usually designed to sit on top of a desk or table. Because the timing and length of exposure are crucial in the successful treatment of various conditions, light therapy requires guidance by a trained professional.

In case you're wondering, turning on the fluorescent or incandescent overhead lights do not count as sun exposure or light therapy; indoor lights are not bright enough. Tanning booths do not count either because your eyes are closed. To increase serotonin levels and get the benefit of light, the rays have to enter through the iris of your eyes. Again, appropriate medical supervision is needed to prevent any eye damage potentially caused by bright light.

Hydrotherapy

Let the sun rejuvenate you by day, and take advantage of the soothing quality of water at night. Hot tubs, bubble baths, pools, and natural hot springs release endorphins, relax muscles, and dilate blood vessels. If you are fortunate enough to live near natural hot springs, the high mineral content gives you a sense of weightlessness while the carbon dioxide forms tiny bubbles on your skin. One of my clients had the perfect analogy when she said, "I feel like I'm floating in a pool of champagne."

Aromatherapy

How do you feel after taking a whiff of a fragrant bouquet of flowers? Or walking by a lilac bush in full bloom? Certain smells relax us; others energize us. Lavender, rosemary, and rose are particularly relaxing, and many bath oils, soaps, lotions, and potpourris contain these and other pleasing scents. Aromatherapy is now receiving validation in scientific literature. The medical journal *Lancet* recently reported that lavender reduced insomnia as much as medication, and another study found that rosemary helped block pain by increasing endorphin levels in the brain.

Until more is known about the health benefits of specific scents, let your nose be your guide. Buy your favorite flowers, light a scented candle, add scented bath oil to your tub of hot water—and combine aromatherapy and hydrotherapy for the ultimate de-stressor.

Acupuncture, Acupressure, and Herbs

China has been privy to the healing qualities of needles, pressure points, and herbs for over five thousand years, but we're just starting to acknowledge their amazing actions. Acupuncture and acupressure have been found to release endorphins, decrease pain sensitivity, and increase blood and energy flow to targeted organs. A number of herbs now have proven medicinal properties and healing power. The following herbs have undergone some of the rigors of scientific testing and are acknowledged to be of potential help to menopausal women:

HERB	BENEFICIAL EFFECT
ginseng	decreases fatigue, estrogenlike effect on the body and brain
valerian root	reduces insomnia, anxiety, and mood swings; has been used as a sedative in Europe for over one thousand years
motherwort	decreases mood swings during PMS and menopause; means "medicinal plant for mother"
St. John's wort	relieves mild depression by increasing serotonin
dong quai	contains phytoestrogens, eases menopausal symptoms
black cohosh	reduces headaches, acts as a mild estrogen

chamomile	calming effect, reduces anxiety
sulfur	reduces hot flashes
ginkgo biloba	dilates blood vessels, increases memory and concentration
chaste berry	reduces hot flashes, night sweats, and vaginal dryness

I've had clients who were disappointed when they felt no different after giving herbs a try. I've had others who reported immense benefits. Individual differences may have to do with different physiologies and different philosophies. Remember the placebo effect: **believing that something will help is half the benefit.**

Herbal medicine is relatively new to this country and has not been subjected to the same testing protocols and quality control standards as drugs. Many women think herbs are harmless—just another form of food. Herbs are plants, but they are not food. In fact, herbs act more like diluted drugs in our bodies, and therefore, they are not without potential risks and side effects. If you do decide to experiment with herbs, be cautious, get guidance from someone who has extensive knowledge, and keep the following in mind:

- Some herbs may produce detrimental effects; even a few deaths have been attributed to herbs. The FDA and American Herbal Products Association now have lists of herbs to avoid: comfrey, ephedra, chaparral, buckthorn, and sassafras are among them.

- Interactions with other herbs, drugs, and nutrients are virtually unknown—buy products that list all the ingredients.

- Don't take any herb every day; the effects are cumulative.

- Don't take more than the recommended dose on the label. More is not better when it comes to herbs.

- Herbs are rarely replacements for drugs, but options to supplement mainstream treatments.

- Inform yourself—read books such as *The Honest Herbal* by Varro Tyler.

- Inform your physician. Beth Israel Hospital in Boston found that 72 percent of those who pursue the more unconventional therapies such as herbs do not share their decision with their physician.

- Don't believe exaggerated claims that herbs (or any other pill or potion) will "treat" menopause, "cure" disease, or "guarantee" health and longevity.

As more people are experimenting with herbs, supplements, and other alternative therapies, more health food companies, multilevel marketing corporations, and self-help books are making exaggerated claims to persuade us that various "miracle" pills can do it all: treat menopause, stop aging, prevent disease, burn fat, boost energy, ward off wrinkles, vanish varicose veins, regrow hair, enhance your sex life, and increase your longevity. There's traditional medicine; there's alternative medicine—then there's pure quackery. When it comes to menopausal remedies, love potions, fatigue-fighting formulas, and "youth-in-a-pill" concoctions the best advice is old advice: *Buyer Beware.*

If you want to live longer, wear your seat belt. If you want to live well, wear your sneakers and a smile. Fitness and happiness will have a more positive impact on your well-being than anything else.

THE PURSUIT OF HORMONAL HAPPINESS

Happiness, contentment, satisfaction—they're what we all strive for. But when changing hormones produce fatigue, mood swings, insomnia, and decreased brain chemicals, these virtues seem out of our reach.

I've had clients ask, "If I go on hormone replacement therapy, will I be happy again?" Maybe and maybe not. Some women feel great on hormone replacement therapy; others feel worse instead of better. Some women take hormones to decrease heart disease and osteoporosis; others avoid them because of breast cancer, gallbladder disease, liver problems, asthma, migraines, and weight gain.

To be or not to be on HRT—that is the question. The problem is, there is no concrete answer. Estrogen does have some amazing effects on the brain, increasing the feel-good brain chemicals serotonin and the endorphins, improving short-term memory, and even reducing the risk of Alzheimer's disease. Estrogen also helps to deposit calcium in our bones and reduces heart disease risk by keeping our HDL levels high and our arteries clean. But hormone replacement does not necessarily guarantee health and happiness or "make us feel ourselves again" as the ads say. Real risks accompany the benefits, and breast cancer terrifies women more than any other potential risk.

The jury is still out on the relationship between hormone replacement and breast cancer. Until a consensus is reached on what estrogen does and doesn't do, each of us needs to make our own decision based on how we feel, our risk profile, and how our bodies react. We may decide to try nothing, try a different dose, try a different combination (sometimes adding a little testosterone does the trick), or try the more natural sources of hormones. A number of pharmacies manufacture hormonal creams, pills, and suppositories made from wild Mexican yams or soy. The initial research on these food-based products is encouraging, giving women another option for hormone replacement as they come to their own decision on the estrogen question.

Hormone replacement may or may not be your lifestyle choice, but happiness can and should be a part of everyone's life. Unfortunately, it's not. A recent study shared some dismal news: Half of menopausal women surveyed said that they felt sad more often than they felt happy. I was recently saddened when one of my clients said, "I try not to be happy, smile, or laugh. I don't want to get deeper laugh lines and wrinkles."

Laughter makes you younger, not older. It releases tension, boosts metabolism, stimulates the immune system, and triggers endorphin and serotonin release. When was the last time you laughed so hard you cried? How did you feel afterward? When was the last time you got the giggles in an inappropriate place? Laughter is fun, silly, therapeutic, and life enhancing.

Some women get their laughs from comedy clubs; others read the comics, find jokes on the Internet, go to the movies (or rent the old comedy classics), watch the funnier sitcoms, browse the card shop (I do it all the time; some cards available now are hilarious), or frequent the humor section of bookstores. You'd be surprised by the number of books whose only goal is to make us laugh. **We're hungry for humor!**

I know of three books written specifically on menopausal humor (that sounds like an oxymoron, but it doesn't have to be): *Menopaws* by Martha Sacks offers an amusing look at menopause from a cat's perspective, *The Noisy Passage: Baby Boomers Do Menopause* by Marie Evans and Ann Shakeshaft provides comic relief as we speed down the hormonal superhighway, and *Living Somewhere Between Estrogen and Death* by Barbara Johnson is filled with many clever quips that she calls "wrinkle busters." Here are a few to entice you:

- You know you're getting older when "Happy Hour" is a nap.
- Growing old is inevitable, growing up is optional.
- It's easy to go for the burn—just sit around and wait for a hot flash.
- You may be older today than you have ever been before, but you are younger than you'll ever be again.
- Being tickled to death is a great way to live. Jumping for joy is good exercise.

Happiness isn't just about laughing. Joy, delight, pleasure, contentment, and satisfaction are all components of happiness. If these are lacking in your life, you have to take charge and add activities that make you feel good. Take a moment and think of ten things that make you smile, feel content, or soothe your soul.

1. _____
2. _____
3. _____
4. _____
5. _____
6. _____
7. _____
8. _____
9. _____
10. _____

Was this list difficult? Did you draw a blank? When I asked Sophia what made her happy, the only thing she could think of was losing weight. Many women think that when they lose weight, they'll finally be happy. Actually, the reverse is true: When you are happy with who you are and what you do, then you'll finally lose weight. You're more active when you're happy, have a faster metabolism (smiling burns more calories than frowning, and laughing burns more calories than walking), and are too busy having fun to overeat. **Happiness is a natural appetite suppressant.**

Another difficulty women have in compiling this list is that they've forgotten what makes them happy. They are spending so much time making everyone else happy that it's been years since they've thought about their own joy. Or, they've become so dependent on others to make them happy that they're at a loss about how to make themselves feel good. To become your own source of contentment, Alice Domar, author of *Healing Mind, Healthy Body*, recommends delivering a message to your conscious and unconscious mind: "I can take care of my needs, and I can feel good about myself without anyone else's confirmation." It's an important message. Say it right now, hand deliver it to your mind, and follow through by doing something that feels good and takes care of your need to be happy.

If you had difficulty with your happiness list, some of the suggestions in this chapter may give you ideas, such as getting a massage (or a facial or a manicure), taking a bath, deep breathing, buying flowers, or just having some quiet time. Happiness is very personal; but women share a number of common ways to bring pleasure to their lives. Survey after survey has found that women rate the following as their major sources of pleasure: eating chocolate (no surprise), getting a massage, getting together with friends, going shopping, and having sex.

Speaking of sex, according to an *American Health* magazine survey, women age 35 to 55 who have the healthiest lifestyles also have the happiest sex lives. Sixty-two percent of the women who describe their health as good report that sex has improved with age. If you haven't experienced this pleasurable boost in intimacy, it may be because of decreased lubrication and a lower sex drive that can accompany menopause. Creams and jellies can help with the lubrication, and The Meno-Positive Approach can help with the lust. Feeling good about yourself spills over to your sex life.

This wasn't enough for Mary Pat. She was in search of an aphrodisiac and asked me if oysters or any other food fit the bill. I told her, "I don't personally know of any research identifying proven aphrodisiacs, but it doesn't hurt to experiment, and please call me when you find one."

To be as healthy as you possibly can during your midlife years—for your sex life, social life, family life, and work life—I would be remiss if I didn't remind you of some important medical tests. No one is happy to find that they have a medical problem, but we are thankful when we catch it early enough to do something about it.

YOUR MIDLIFE CHECKUP

"All of a sudden, I feel mortal. When I don't get enough sleep, I feel wiped out. When I drink too much alcohol, I feel horrible. When I don't eat a variety of healthy foods, I feel weak and malnourished. I never really thought about my health until my 40th birthday, but when I reached the midlife marker, I had a renewed commitment to take care of myself."

Many women experience this client's type of renewed commitment to health. During the midlife years, we become more aware of what makes us feel good and what doesn't, and we start paying more attention to our health needs. One way to focus on your health is to practice prevention by scheduling an appointment for some important medical tests. Those most important for midlife women include:

- **Breast exam.** A professional breast exam is recommended every year. One extensive study found that 40 percent of all women over age 40 hadn't had a professional breast exam in the past year. Are you one of them?

- **Mammogram.** Despite the recent controversy on when and how often mammograms should be done, most health professionals still recommend a baseline mammogram by age 40, every other year in our forties, and every year after age 50. Mammography may not be the perfect screening tool, but it's the best we have to detect small tumors that breast self-exams can't find.

- **Pap smear.** Annual testing is advised for all women. Since pap smears were instituted in the 1940s, deaths from cervical cancer have dropped 40 percent! Early detection saves lives.

- **Blood pressure screening.** Every other year is recommended; if you are African American, you have a higher risk for hypertension and should be screened every year.

- **Cholesterol testing.** Have your blood cholesterol checked at least every five years and make sure you have a full lipid panel that measures LDL (the bad) cholesterol, HDL (the good) cholesterol, and triglycerides. As estrogen decreases during the transition, HDLs decrease and LDLs increase. Heart disease is the leading cause of death for women, killing ten times more women than breast cancer.

- **Skin cancer screening.** After age 40, your risk of melanoma increases and annual screening is advised. You may use sunscreen now, but think of the sunburns you got as a child, teenager, and young adult.

- **Colon cancer screening.** The sigmoidoscopy may not be our favorite medical test, but it's a necessity at age 50. Colon cancer is on the rise for women, and the risk increases as we grow older.

- **Bone density testing.** Health professionals recommend that all women have a bone density test when they stop menstruating. Some are also urging a baseline bone scan at age 35, so that when you're tested again after the transition, you'll know how much bone you've lost, if any. And you can use this information as you're weighing the decision whether or not to take HRT.

- **Thyroid screening.** More and more health professionals are recognizing the importance of periodic thyroid screening for women between the ages of 35 and 60. Johns Hopkins researchers did a cost-effective analysis and concluded that it makes sense from a financial standpoint to screen women starting at age 35. A blood test of thyroid levels costs only $30 to $50, but the cost of repeated visits to find the source of malaise and our troubles can reach thousands.

Thyroid screening may be the one medical test that you haven't heard of yet. Most women are not aware that thyroid activity (the gland that determines our metabolism) diminishes during menopause, and an underactive thyroid can lead to an overwhelming menopausal experience.

An estimated 4 million of us are walking around with a sluggish thyroid, and most of them are 35- to 55-year-old women who don't know it. The symptoms of hypothyroidism (low thyroid) are similar to the signs of menopause: fatigue, hair loss, dry skin, muscle and joint pain, weight gain, depression, and forgetfulness. Your doctor may tell you that you are "just menopausal," under too much stress, or suffering from depression. He or she might say, "Try HRT, try Prozac, try exercise, try slowing down. You're getting older."

But what one in five women might need to try is thyroid replacement. Giving your body the thyroid it needs may make all the difference in the world, helping with energy, moods, and weight loss. Thyroid medication may increase the risk for osteoporosis, so if you find that your thyroid needs a boost, never take more than your prescribed dose and give extra care to your bones with diet and exercise.

Whether it be with medical tests, mindfulness skills, or education—the more you know about your body and health, the more equipped you'll be to journey through menopause consciously. Continue to nurture a growing sense of understanding of your body, and use that understanding to grow healthier, happier, and stronger every day.

LIFESTYLES OF THE RELAXED AND FEARLESS

Menopause is our wake-up call, the body's way of getting our attention to take care of ourselves for the rest of our lives. That may mean reducing stress, losing excess weight, exercising four days a week, eating more vegetables, meditating, putting up a Do Not Disturb sign, focusing on what makes you happy, taking herbs, taking hormones, taking thryroid, or taking the time to get important medical tests. As you live a more positive lifestyle and become more connected with your needs, you may also find that you have a greater need to speak your mind, share your opinions, and start acting out of intuition instead of cultural norms.

As one of my more verbal clients said, "Basically, I don't take s—t from anyone anymore. I finally speak up and trust my feelings. I have more confidence in myself and my abilities. Things I put up with for years I just don't do anymore. I thank menopause for that."

Menopause can be a time when we no longer question who we are, what we want, and how to get it. We become stronger in our convictions and more self-assured in our purpose. This revelation is evident in the menopausal insights women have shared with me:

- "I now look life straight in the eye to decide what's worth my time and what isn't."

- "I've stopped worrying about what other people think and only worry what I think."

- "My needs have always come last, but now I realize that putting my needs first isn't selfish, it's immensely satisfying."

- "Menopause is like cleaning out my life's closet, throwing out old fears, restrictions, and insecurities."

- "Menopause has been my catalyst for more open, honest communication with my partner, family, friends, doctors, and coworkers."

- "Instead of thinking I don't have time to take care of myself, I now realize that I can't afford not to take care of myself."

- "I'm older, and I can't say I'm happy about it. But I'd never trade in this 45-year-old brain for a 25-year-old body."

- "I feel lighter because I've removed the unnecessary baggage from my life including people, commitments, and obligations. I finally have the guts to say 'no' to things I don't want to do."

- "I'm glad I'm in menopause. I'm more confident, and people take me more seriously. I'm celebrating because I finally feel like I've grown up."

Women in other cultures have always celebrated menopause and looked forward to this transformation to mature adulthood. Japanese women view menopause as freedom from reproduction and greater independence. In Celtic cultures, the young woman is the flower, the mother the fruit, and the elder woman the seed containing all the knowledge of the other parts. In Native American cultures, older women are considered wiser because they retain their "wise blood."

Women do gain more wisdom, insight, knowledge, freedom, and independence during the midlife years, and it's time our society recognized these attributes too. Menopause is just the beginning of this positive transformation. As hormone levels rebalance, hot flashes recede, and fat cells retreat, we enter a new place in our lives—the best yet.

HOW WILL YOU LIVE A MENO-POSITIVE LIFESTYLE?

As with everything I have presented in this book, what I have covered in this chapter are lifestyle options—informing you of what you can do to take responsibility for your well-being, reduce stress, increase happiness, and manage your weight. The choice, as always, is yours.

- ❏ I will make it a priority to take care of my body.
- ❏ I will think "less stress" for a healthier menopause.
- ❏ I will give myself some quiet time to silence my stress response.
- ❏ I will use imagery to take mini mind vacations.
- ❏ When I'm obsessing about something, I will ask, "Is this going to matter a year from now?"
- ❏ I will "live in the moment" by being aware of what's going on and what I'm feeling.
- ❏ I will experiment with mind-body techniques such as massage, meditation, and deep breathing.
- ❏ I will step out in the sun for fifteen minutes to increase serotonin.
- ❏ I will take advantage of the soothing quality of water with baths, pools, and hot tubs.
- ❏ I will use my sense of smell to relax and rejuvenate.
- ❏ I will become more informed about herbs and inform my doctor if I experiment with them.
- ❏ I will beware of pills and potions with exaggerated claims and false promises.
- ❏ I will carefully weigh the decision of whether or not to take hormone replacement therapy.
- ❏ I will laugh, smile, and add activities that bring joy to my life.
- ❏ I will make an appointment to get the necessary screening tests for midlife women.
- ❏ I will think of menopause as an opportunity to become stronger, more self-assured, and more vocal.
- ❏ I will turn the page and read the last chapter to fully outsmart my fat cells during menopause—and beyond.

chapter nine

IT'S NOT OVER TILL THE
FAT CELL SINGS

You may be nearing the end of this book, but your commitment to outsmarting your midlife fat cells has just begun. I have shared everything there is to know about stubborn menopausal weight gain, and everything within your power to manage it. But "everything" can't happen overnight, over a week, or even over a month. The Meno-Positive Approach takes time.

How much time? The most accurate answer is: a lifetime. It takes most women about six to twelve months to outsmart their midlife fat cells, but it takes a lifetime to keep them that way. Please don't let this answer trigger a reflex to close the book and rush back to the store for one that says "how to get your 20-year-old body back in twenty days." You now know better: a 20-year-old body is only for 20-year-olds, and given our busy, time-consuming schedules, twenty days is barely enough time to read any book—never mind recondition our fat cells.

It may take months to change the way your fat cells function so that they store less and release more, but it only takes minutes to receive the initial benefits of The Meno-Positive Approach. In fact, from the moment you started reading chapter 1, you experienced the first level of benefits: knowledge. What you'll continue to get out of this approach is best described as a pyramid with three distinct levels.

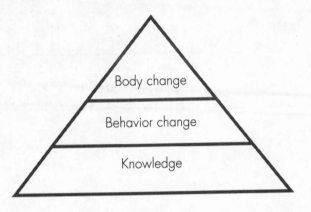

Even if you choose to go no further with The Meno-Positive Approach, you'll always know:

1. why your clothes are tighter in the waist
2. why you're gaining weight even though you're eating less
3. why your exercise program isn't working like it used to
4. why your menopausal fat cells are growing and multiplying
5. why dieting will only cause more weight gain

Your fat cells (especially those in your waist) are responding to lower estrogen levels, a drop in metabolism, and a biological need to maintain your physical and emotional health. You can't fight your midlife fat cells with dieting. They will only fight back with more force.

Because you have this vital information tucked away in your brain, you'll always have a better understanding of your body. But why stop here? Even greater benefits are right around the corner. As you begin to put The Meno-Positive Approach into practice over the next few weeks, the second level of benefits will surface: behavior change. You used to eat two meals a day, but now you're automatically eating five smaller meals. Your hand weights used to be buried underneath the bed, but now they are beside your bed and used twice a week. You'll wake up one day in the not too distant future realizing that:

1. you haven't even thought about dieting or getting on the scale
2. you've exercised consistently for weeks with a variety of different activities—and it wasn't nearly as torturous as you thought
3. you've become an instinctive eater by responding to your hunger and fullness levels
4. you've made conscious food choices that will help balance your body during the transition
5. you've taken care of your body and mind by reducing stress and enhancing relaxation—and people are willing to give you space for some quiet time

These positive behavior changes will make a noticeable difference in how you feel each day. You'll feel more in tune with your body because of greater internal awareness; you'll feel lighter because you won't be weighed down by dieting and body dissatisfaction; and you'll feel less tension, fewer mood swings, and more energy because your body is more balanced.

As your behaviors continue to change over the next few months, you'll achieve the number one goal of every midlife woman: measurable body changes. But this time (as opposed to past dieting) you'll accomplish these changes with a natural, female-oriented, permanent approach, and you'll feel confident when you discover that:

1. you've stopped gaining weight or have lost weight
2. you've gained muscle mass
3. your muscles are more toned and stronger

4. your clothes are fitting more comfortably
5. you've reached a healthy midlife weight and your fat cells are singing

You may faintly hear them humming "I Did It My Way" because you've allowed them to grow some and fulfill their menopausal duty, but didn't overstimulate their growth with dieting and overeating. Fat cells want to grow by 20 percent not 200 percent. They don't want to cause too much weight gain because they don't want you (and therefore them) to have orthopedic problems, chronic diseases, or a shorter lifespan. Fat cells are trying to keep you healthy. They want to live a long, active life too.

How will you know when your fat cells are singing? How will you know when they've been outsmarted? You can have your body fat analyzed periodically to measure changes in fat lost and muscle gained, and when you reach a plateau, you'll know your fat cells have shrunk as much as they can without compromising your well-being. Or, you can simply trust that your body will stabilize on its own and will give you a thumbs up sign when it's reached a comfortable, healthy weight.

WHAT DOES A HEATHY MIDLIFE WOMAN LOOK LIKE?

If we look to Hollywood for that vision, we see Goldie Hawn, Jane Fonda, Lauren Hutton, Dolly Parton, Ivana Trump, and the like telling us that 50 is fabulous in their slim-fitting designer outfits. A few women do naturally travel through menopause without visible changes, but many mask their changes with plastic surgery—a sculpt here, a tuck there, and liposuction everywhere.

Instead of looking to fashion magazines or movie screens for an image of what's realistic and healthy, look to your neighborhood, your office, your hair salon, your grocery store, your friends, and your family. Healthy midlife women are everywhere. They are ordinary women who exercise, don't diet, and eat instinctively. They are women who move freely and feel comfortable in their maturing bodies. Some spotlight celebrities do fit the bill: Raquel Welch, Meryl Streep, Diane Keaton, Whoopi Goldberg, Jessica Lange, and Cybill Shepherd come to mind. They've gained some weight, but not a lot. Sophia Loren is known to be especially proud of her ample curves and is famous for saying "Everything you see I owe to spaghetti." Now, who's saying that pasta makes you fat? If that's the kind of fat it makes you, I'm having spaghetti tonight and every night.

Curves, straight lines, high-waisted, low-waisted, no waist—a variety of different shapes and weights is healthy. Many factors, including age, genetics, metabolism, bone structure, musculature, and body type, affect how much weight we carry and where we carry it. We are each biologically unique, and therefore, we each have a different weight that is optimal and healthy for us. Your doctor, your scale, your aerobics instructor, or the height/weight charts can't tell you what you should weigh. Nobody can because only your body knows for sure. If you are exercising and fueling your body with instinctive eating habits, and your body gravitates to a certain weight—and feels comfortable there—then that's *your healthy midlife weight.*

But like most of my clients, you probably want specifics, so here they are. The average healthy menopausal woman weighs 145 pounds, has a body fat percentage of 32 percent, carries 98 pounds of muscle, wears a size 10, and has a 28½-inch waist. Now that I've given you the numbers, I don't want you to compare yourself to them, unless you're exactly 5 feet 4 inches tall and have a medium frame. You may not be anywhere close to the average—you may be 6 feet tall or 5 feet tall, small boned or large boned. If you fall outside of the norm, you're not average—you're exceptional!

For those of you who are exceptional, here are some other characteristics that describe healthy weight women.

A HEALTHY MIDLIFE WOMAN   DO YOU?

	YES	NO
1. Walks up three flights of stairs without getting out of breath	____	____
2. Has a clean bill of health without weight-related problems such as high blood pressure, high blood cholesterol, or adult-onset diabetes	____	____
3. Wears a bathing suit in public	____	____
4. Wears a size larger than she did ten years ago	____	____
5. Has defined muscles	____	____
6. Nourishes her body	____	____
7. Moves her body at least four days a week	____	____
8. Looks in the mirror and says "Yes!" (instead of "Yuck!")	____	____
9. Carries two to ten more pounds than she did ten years ago	____	____
10. Has some cellulite on the backs of her thighs	____	____
11. Has a waist that's 1 to 2 inches larger than ten years ago	____	____
12. Has a body fat percentage between 25 percent and 35 percent (If you haven't had your body composition tested, you will not know the answer to this.)	____	____

If you answered "yes" to these questions, no matter what you weigh, you are at a weight that is healthy for *you*—and The Meno-Positive Approach will keep you there. If you answered "no" to any, most, or all of these questions, you haven't yet out-smarted your midlife fat cells—and The Meno-Positive Approach will get you there. That may mean losing five pounds or fifty pounds of excess weight caused by underexercising and overeating. Or that may mean getting fit by gaining a few pounds of muscle and keeping your weight stable.

Regardless of how close or far you are from achieving a healthy midlife weight, remember: This is a process that takes time. You can't push a fast-forward button to gain muscle, you can't force your fat cells to release fat, and you can't let the "I want it yesterday" attitude get in the way. **You've got to stick with it to trick your fat cells.**

PATIENCE, PERSEVERANCE, PERSPECTIVE

"I don't think I can do it. I can't wait months for change. I have to get this weight off right now. Don't you have something that will burn fat as I sleep so I can wake up tomorrow trimmer and thinner?" If, like this woman, you don't think that you have the patience to work with your fat cells for permanent change, consider other times in your life when something has been so important to you that you toughed it out. Many of us have done it with education, raising children, making a marriage work, starting a business, publishing a book, or fighting for a political issue we believe in. Achieving a healthy weight is important to you, too, and you can find the patience to accomplish this goal with The Meno-Positive Approach.

Patience is "the capacity to hold steadfast despite diffi-culty." Managing midlife weight gain is not easy (and don't believe anyone who says it is). Fitting exercise into an already overbooked schedule is a challenge. Resisting the temptation to diet is hard work—especially if your high school reunion, son's wedding, or other important event is coming up. Anticipate these and other potential difficulties, hold your course, and *fight fat with fortitude.*

Perseverance is "persistence in the face of opposition." Sometimes you may feel like the whole world is against you. Society advocates restriction, thinness, and quick fixes; your doctor may try to persuade you to go on some diet plan; your friend may encourage you to take a fat-burning pill. *Don't do it!* Persevere with the instinctive eating approach and a diet-free lifestyle—and endure with exercise.

I have to take this opportunity to give exercise one more plug. If you only get one message from this book—*exercise!* If you don't exercise, you won't manage midlife weight gain. It's that simple. If you don't exercise aerobically for four hours a week, you won't lose fat. If you don't strength-train for one hour a week, you won't stimulate your metabolism and rebuild muscle.

But don't think that exercise (or anything else) will guarantee a changeless, timeless body. The National Runner's Health Survey found that we'd have to run fifty-two miles a week (that's two marathons!) to fit into our college jeans. The moral of this study: You can't run away from midlife weight gain.

Perspective is "the capacity to view things clearly." If a week goes by and you haven't exercised, it doesn't mean you've blown it. A week is insignificant in the context of the rest of your life. Just pick a day to start again. If you overeat at dinner tonight, you will not gain five pounds by morning. Just be extra aware of your hunger and fullness signals tomorrow. "Two steps forward, one step back" is a normal part of the change process. If you didn't take a step back every now and then, I'd be worried that you were turning this approach into a diet and trying to be perfect.

Perfection doesn't exist in The Meno-Positive Approach because there is no right or wrong way of eating, exercising, or living. Expect setbacks, learn from your experiences, use your common sense, and keep your motivation high with two other suggestions:

1. Acknowledge your changes no matter how small.
2. Take on some new midlife mottos.

First, let's talk about patting yourself on the back. Even on one morning bypassing the scale is an achievement. Eating a smaller dinner on one night is a commendable change. Going for a walk on one afternoon is an accomplishment. And all of these seemingly little changes add up to big changes in your body.

I've had clients who were discouraged because they thought this approach wasn't working for them. Mira comes to mind as an example. After two months of making commendable strides in her exercise program and eating habits, she noticed little change in her body and was ready to throw in the towel. But after completing the following questionnaire, she realized that she had changed dramatically. This acknowledgment gave her the stick-to-itiveness she needed to continue for another three months until her body changed significantly.

I recommend that you take this questionnaire every month or so during your change process. Because simple yes/no answers with their black or white verdicts are too limiting, I have designed a rating scale from 1 to 5 so that you can track your successful progression through each of the principles of The Meno-Positive Approach to a Trimmer Transition.

1—no change, haven't done a thing, I've been avoiding it, I'm in denial

2 through 4—I'm trying, I did it once, I'm doing it some of the time, I'm doing it most of the time, I'm getting there

5—I did it, I've changed, I never think about dieting anymore, I'm consistent with exercise, I'm managing stress

	NO	GETTING THERE	YES

PRINCIPLE 1: ACQUIRING MENO-POSITIVE ATTITUDES

	NO		GETTING THERE		YES
Have you given up dieting?	1	2	3	4	5
Have you given up the scale?	1	2	3	4	5
Do you have a greater acceptance of your body?	1	2	3	4	5
Do you have a greater acceptance of menopause?	1	2	3	4	5

PRINCIPLE 2: MASTERING MENO-POSITIVE FITNESS

	NO		GETTING THERE		YES
Are you exercising aerobically 4 hours a week?	1	2	3	4	5
Are you strength-training 1 hour a week?	1	2	3	4	5
Are you doing weight-bearing exercises?	1	2	3	4	5
Are you doing a variety of different activities?	1	2	3	4	5

	NO	**GETTING THERE**			**YES**

PRINCIPLE 3: EMBRACING
MENO-POSITIVE EATING HABITS

Are you responding to your signals of hunger and fullness?	1	2	3	4	5
Are you eating smaller, more frequent meals?	1	2	3	4	5
Are your dinner meals smaller?	1	2	3	4	5
Are you eating your favorite foods?	1	2	3	4	5

PRINCIPLE 4: MAXIMIZING
MENO-POSITIVE FOOD CHOICES

Are you responding to your food cravings?	1	2	3	4	5
Are you eating your phytoestrogens?	1	2	3	4	5
Are you eating 5 servings of fruits and vegetables a day?	1	2	3	4	5
Are you drinking water throughout the day?	1	2	3	4	5
Are you eating 2 servings of protein a day?	1	2	3	4	5
Are you consuming enough calcium?	1	2	3	4	5

PRINCIPLE 5: LIVING A
MENO-POSITIVE LIFESTYLE

Are you managing your stress?	1	2	3	4	5
Are you taking the time to relax, unwind, and rejuvenate?	1	2	3	4	5
Are you giving yourself some peace and quiet?	1	2	3	4	5
Are you practicing mind-body techniques?	1	2	3	4	5

	NO	GETTING THERE		YES
Are you scheduling activities that make you happy?	1	2 3	4	5
Are you scheduling the important midlife medical tests?	1	2 3	4	5
Are you speaking your mind, sharing your opinions, and saying "no" to the things you don't want to do?	1	2 3	4	5

(Each time you take this questionnaire, use a different color pen or marking symbol so that you can visually follow your timeline of successful behavior change.)

You can also use this questionnaire to identify what you need to focus on in the future. Maybe you've done great enhancing your eating habits, but have all 1s on the exercise questions. Perhaps you've concentrated on maximizing your food choices, but have purposefully put off listening to your hunger and fullness signals. Go back to pages 97, 131, 157, 187, and 215, photocopy or tear out the "How Will You . . . " worksheets for each of the principles of The Meno-Positive Approach, recommit to the strategies that made sense to you when you first read the chapters, have the belief that behavior change will lead to body change, and have the patience to wait until your fat cells sing.

While you're patiently waiting, you can also skim through the book again and highlight key phrases and passages that will serve as your midlife motivational mottos. But if you don't have the time (because you're now exercising and getting weekly massages), I've done the work for you. Here are the top twenty-five inspirational phrases to keep you on track.

1. Menopause is not a disease to be treated; it's a transition to be experienced.

2. *You* are not gaining weight; your menopausal *body* is.

3. Fat cells are your menopausal helper, coming to your aid to produce estrogen for you.

4. Dieting causes megamenopause and more midlife weight gain.

5. Dieting thins your hair, skin, bones, and thinking. Dieting thins everything but *you*.

6. Some midlife weight gain is healthy—and fitness, not fatness, is the key to a long life.

7. Throw away your scale, but not your common sense.

8. Who you are is more important than what you weigh.

9. Focus on muscle gain, not fat loss.

10. Exercise combats menopausal fat.

11. To master menopausal fitness, you need both aerobics and strength training.

12. Don't diet, eat! Don't eat less, move more! Don't eat less frequently, eat more often!

13. *What* you eat is not as important as *how much* you eat.

14. A handful of food will fill your stomach without overfilling it.

15. Physical hunger is when your body needs nourishment; emotional hunger is when your soul needs nourishment.

16. Midlife women need to eat midmorning, midday, and midafternoon.

17. Carbohydrates, fat, and protein are your "feel good" foods that will boost your "feel good" brain chemicals.

18. Chocolate is your menopausal mood stabilizer.

19. Your menopausal body can't function well on a staple of fat-free foods.

20. Phytoestrogens fight fat cells.

21. Outwitting stress is an effective way to outsmart midlife fat cells.

22. Happiness is a natural appetite suppressant.

23. You've got to stick with it to trick your fat cells.

24. Your body will find its own healthy midlife weight.

25. You have more healthy wisdom in your body than all the medical libraries in the world.

If you are just entering the menopausal transition, you have a decade or more to keep your motivation high with these midlife mottos and the other suggestions in this chapter. If you are nearing the end of this fascinating female passage, you probably wish I had written this book ten years ago. Don't despair, you still have plenty of time to tame your midlife fat cells. Regardless of where you are in the transition, I guarantee you that menopause will end, your weight gain will stop, and you'll feel revitalized.

WHEN THE TRANSITION IS OVER

When you enter your postmenopausal years, moods even out, thinking clears, sleep patterns improve, energy returns, and fat cells retreat. After working overtime for the past decade, your fat cells look forward to retirement and actually release some fat on their own recognizance. The fat cells in your thighs shrink the most (hallelujah!), and those in your buttocks, waist, arms, and cheeks get a bit smaller too. The only fat cells that continue working and growing are those in your breasts. Thinner thighs, larger breasts—maybe now you'll look forward to your post-menopausal years!

The years following menopause will most likely be very different from the years preceding it. Like a fine red wine, we get better and better over time. Here are some other transformations to look forward to:

- You'll no longer accelerate the greenhouse effect with your hot flashes (although 1 percent say their hot flashes last forever).

- You'll realize that your husband or significant other isn't such a jerk after all.

- You'll find the five sets of keys you lost over the last ten years.

- You'll look at your younger friends going through the transition and think "was my menopause that bad?" Yes, it probably was, but now it doesn't really matter because you feel great. Those women who report the most difficulty during the transition feel the best two years after it's over.

- Your weight frustrations and food preoccupations don't seem to matter anymore either. When you were in the transition, they consumed your life. Now that you're out of it, they almost seem silly.

WHEN YOU'RE IN IT	WHEN IT'S OVER
you weigh yourself	you start weighing your priorities
you're worried about fat plumping out your stomach	you want fat to plump out your wrinkles
you fight your hunger	you fight against world hunger
you strive for thinness	you speak out against thinness
your free time is spent at weight loss centers	your free time is spent volunteering at rape crisis centers
you fear hip expansion	you fear hip replacement
losing weight is your goal	living well is your goal

The benefits of The Meno-Positive Approach don't stop when you stop menstruating. They continue to help your bones, mind, and general health when you're 60, 80, even 100 years old. *American Health* magazine recently interviewed centenarians on their secrets to a long life. Gender was the dominant factor, with the vast majority of all those a hundred and over being women, but they also found that an active life, a positive attitude, and an occasional chocolate chip cookie deserved much of the credit. These women didn't restrict their fat and sugar intake, and they weren't affected by the thinness craze and the dieting industry as we have been. When the dieting epidemic started in the 1960s, they were in their 60s, already postmenopausal, unconcerned about losing weight, and unaffected by the restrictive and dangerous culture of dieting. In addition to a positive attitude and active lifestyle, **maybe a diet-free way of life is also one of their longevity secrets.**

We can learn a great deal from these wise older women. They maintained a moderate weight and instinctively followed the principles of The Meno-Positive Approach without reading a book or joining a program—and they lived to be a hundred to tell about it.

As you reach your later years, you will realize that you're healthy and strong because you gave up dieting and took care of your body. When you look back, you'll realize that your menopausal fat cells were really doing you a favor.

THANK YOU, FAT CELLS

If fat cells didn't come to the rescue during menopause, you'd have more hot flashes, more bone loss, more hip fractures, more anxiety, more wrinkles, more fatigue, more memory loss—and a shorter life.

If you were a fat cell what would you do? If you could lend a helping hand to live longer, decrease disease risk, supply a natural source of estrogen, and make the transition easier, wouldn't you take advantage of the opportunity by becoming more powerful, larger, and more efficient?

Of course you would, so instead of cursing your midlife fat cells, congratulate them for a job well done. Thank your fat cells for looking out for your health and well-being and apologize to your body for years of dieting and not taking care of it. This moving poem by Marlena Gutierrez may give you some of the words you're searching for.

An Apology to My Body

For all the times I hated you, said you were "too fat," "too ugly," "too" anything.

For all the times I cried in frustration because you didn't look like I wanted you to.

For all the times I put you down in my own mind and in front of others.

For all the times I allowed someone to criticize you and judge you as "not good enough."

For all the times I thought you were awkward, graceless, clumsy.

For all the times I tried to change you by dieting, depriving you of true nourishment.

For all those times, forgive me.

Forgive me for not seeing you as the wondrous and beautiful body you really are and always have been.

Our bodies are wondrous and beautiful in all sizes and at all stages of life. I hope that I have been successful in conveying this message to you. Midlife weight gain is a necessity for female health, as natural and important as the weight we gained in puberty and pregnancy. Menopause is a pivotal stage of female passage, awakening us to new and rewarding ways of living. Form a partnership with your maturing body, embrace its changes, let its wisdom guide you—and experience enhanced health and self-acceptance as you journey through your midlife years and beyond.

Appendix A: Meno-positive Eating Records

If you are the type of person who benefits from some structure and hands-on awareness building, I suggest keeping eating records for as long as you find them helpful. I have included a sample and a blank eating record for you to use as a guideline.

MENO-POSITIVE EATING RECORDS

Time of day	Are you hungry?	Are you craving anything?	What did you eat?	Did you fill your stomach without overfilling it?
6:30 am	a little	a bagel	a bagel with cream cheese	yes
			Coffee	
			orange juice	
9:30 am	Yes	not really	apple	yes
			few pretzels	
12:15 pm	very!	a roast beef Sandwich	1/2 roast beef Sandwich	yes
			lettuce and tomato	
			Swiss cheese	
3:30 pm	a little	chocolate!	2 small pieces of chocolate	yes - I didn't over eat chocolate!
			glass of Soy milk	
6:30 pm	yes	spinach	chicken breast	? feel a little full
			spinach - 1c	
			rice	

Reflect on your day:
Did you eat small, frequent meals? Yes
Did you eat the majority of your food during the day? yes
Did you eat phytoestrogens? yes - Soy milk
Did you eat five servings of fruits and vegetables? yes
Did you eat two servings of protein? yes
Did you consume enough calcium? with supplements - yes
Did you drink water throughout the day? yes - had 5 glasses

MENO-POSITIVE EATING RECORDS

Time of day	Are you hungry?	Are you craving anything?	What did you eat?	Did you fill your stomach without overfilling it?
___	___	___	_____	_____
		___	_____	
			_____	
___	___	___	_____	_____
		___	_____	
			_____	
___	___	___	_____	_____
		___	_____	
			_____	
___	___	___	_____	_____
		___	_____	
			_____	
___	___	___	_____	_____
		___	_____	
			_____	
___	___	___	_____	_____
		___	_____	
		___	_____	
___	___	___	_____	_____
		___	_____	
			_____	

Reflect on your day:
    Did you eat small, frequent meals?
    Did you eat the majority of your food during the day?
    Did you eat phytoestrogens?
    Did you eat five servings of fruits and vegetables?
    Did you eat two servings of protein?
    Did you consume enough calcium?
    Did you drink water throughout the day?

Appendix B: Additional Resources

EATING JOURNALS AND OTHER PUBLICATIONS

For journals, workbooks, and other materials helpful in changing eating and exercise habits, visit the Waterhouse Publications Website at **http://waterpub.nlis.net** or write to:

Waterhouse Publications
P.O. Box 4735
Portland, ME 04112

SEMINARS AND WORKSHOPS

If your organization is interested in a presentation on *Outsmarting the Midlife Fat Cell* or other women's health topics, please contact:

Debra Waterhouse
6114 LaSalle Avenue, #342
Oakland, CA 94611

Appendix C: Suggested Reading

I have attempted to provide a comprehensive reading list on menopause and related topics. Although I may not subscribe to everything the authors recommend, each book has valuable information to offer.

MENOPAUSE

Barbach, L. *The Pause*. New York: Signet, 1993.

Cobb, J. O. *Understanding Menopause*. New York: Penguin, 1994.

Cone, F. K. *Making Sense of Menopause*. New York: Simon & Schuster, 1994.

Evans, M., and A. Shakeshaft. *The Noisy Passage*. Bridgeport, Conn.: Hysteria Publications, 1996.

Ford, G. *Listening to Your Hormones*. Rocklin, Calif.: Prima Publishing, 1996.

Gittleman, A. L. *Super Nutrition for Menopause*. New York: Pocket Books, 1993.

Greenwood, S. *Menopause Naturally*. Volcano, Calif.: Volcano Press, 1992.

Greer, G. *The Change*. New York: Knopf, 1992.

Jacobowitz, R. S. *150 Most-Asked Questions About Menopause*. New York: Hearst Books, 1993.

Johnson, B. *Living Somewhere Between Estrogen and Death*. Dallas, Tex.: Word Publishing, 1997.

Jovanovic, L. with S. Levert. *A Woman Doctor's Guide to Menopause*. New York: Hyperion, 1993.

Landau, C., M. G. Cyr, and A. W. Moulton. *The Complete Book of Menopause*. New York: Perigee, 1994.

Lark, S. *The Estrogen Decision Self Help Book*. Berkeley, Calif.: Celestial Arts, 1995.

Lark, S. *The Menopause Self Help Book*. Berkeley, Calif.: Celestial Arts, 1992.

Laux, M., and C. Conrad. *Natural Woman, Natural Menopause.* New York: HarperCollins, 1997.

Love, S., and K. Lindsey. *Dr. Susan Love's Hormone Book.* New York: Random House, 1997.

Lucks, N., and M. Smith. *A Woman's Midlife Companion.* Rocklin, Calif.: Prima Publishing, 1997.

Maas, P., S. E. Brown, and N. Bruning. *The MEND Clinic Guide to Natural Medicine for Menopause and Beyond.* New York: Dell, 1997.

Marshel, J. E., and L. Konner. *Trouble-Free Menopause.* New York: Avon, 1995.

Moquette-Magee, E. *Eat Well for a Healthy Menopause.* New York: John Wiley & Sons, 1996.

Noteloritz, M., and D. Tonnessen. *Menopause and Midlife Health.* New York: St. Martin's Press, 1994.

Ojeda, L. *Menopause Without Medicine.* Alameda, Calif.: Hunter House, 1995.

Perry, S., and K. O'Hanlan. *Natural Menopause.* Reading, Mass.: Addison-Wesley, 1997.

Sacks, M. *Menopaws.* Berkeley, Calif.: Ten Speed Press, 1995.

Sheehy, G. *The Silent Passage.* New York: Pocket Books, 1993.

Teaff, N. L., and K. W. Wiley. *Perimenopause: Preparing for the Change.* Rocklin, Calif.: Prima Publishing, 1996.

Vliet, E. L. *Screaming to Be Heard: Hormonal Connections Women Suspect and Doctors Ignore.* New York: M. Evans and Co., 1995.

Weed, S. *Menopause: The Wise Woman Way.* Woodstock, N.Y.: Ash Tress, 1992.

COOKBOOKS FOR MENOPAUSE

DeAngelis, L., and M. Siple. *Recipes for Change: Gourmet Whole Food Cooking for Health and Vitality at Menopause.* New York: Dutton, 1996.

Hurley, J. B. *The Good Herb.* New York: William Morrow, 1995.

Luchetti, C. *The Hot Flash Cookbook.* San Francisco: Chronicle Books, 1997.

Shandler, N. *Estrogen: The Natural Way—Over 250 Easy and Delicious Recipes for Menopause*. New York: Villard, 1997.

Winter, R. *Super Soy, The Miracle Bean*. New York: Crown, 1996.

FITNESS

Andes, K. *A Woman's Book of Strength*. New York: Perigee, 1995.

Bailey, C. *Smart Exercise*. New York: Houghton Mifflin, 1994.

Bailey, C., and L. Bishop. *The Fit or Fat Woman*. Boston: Houghton Mifflin, 1989.

Blair, S. N. *Living with Exercise*. Dallas, Tex.: American Health Publishing, 1991.

Birch, B. B. *Power Yoga*. New York: Simon & Schuster, 1995.

Fahey, T. D., and G. Hutchinson. *Weight Training for Women*. Mountain View, Calif.: Mayfield Publishing, 1992.

Evans, W., and I. H. Rosenberg. *Biomarkers: The 10 Determinants of Aging You Can Control*. New York: Simon & Schuster, 1991.

Green, B., and O. Winfrey. *Make the Connection*. New York: Hyperion, 1996.

Mahle, J., and L. Jaffee. *The Bodywise Woman*. Champaign, Ill.: Human Kinetics, 1996.

Nelson, M. *Strong Women Stay Young*. New York: Bantam Books, 1997.

Peterson, J., C. Bryant, C. and S. Peterson. *Strength Training for Women*. Champaign, Ill.: Human Kinetics, 1995.

Rippe, J. M. *Fit Over Forty*. New York: William Morrow, 1996.

GENERAL NUTRITION AND WOMEN'S HEALTH

Carper, J. *Food—Your Miracle Medicine*. New York: HarperCollins, 1993.

Doress-Worters, P. B., and D. L. Siegal. *The New Ourselves, Growing Older*. New York: Simon & Schuster, 1994.

Fletcher, A. *Thin for Life*. Shelburne, Vt.: Chapters Publishing, 1994.

Love, S. *Dr. Susan Love's Breast Book*. Reading, Mass.: Addison-Wesley, 1991.

Mellin, L. *The Solution: Winning Ways to Permanent Weight Loss.* New York: HarperCollins, 1997.

Mitchell, S., and C. Christie. *I'd Kill for a Cookie: A Simple Six-Week Plan to Conquer Stress Eating.* New York: Dutton, 1997.

Northrup, C. *Women's Bodies, Women's Wisdom.* New York: Bantam Books, 1994.

Reichman, J. *I'm Too Young to Get Old.* New York: Times Books, 1996.

Snyderman, N. *Dr. Nancy Snyderman's Guide to Good Health for Women Over Forty.* San Diego: Harcourt Brace, 1996.

Somer, E. *Food and Mood.* New York: Henry Holt, 1995.

Somer, E. *Nutrition for Women.* New York: Henry Holt, 1993.

Stacey, M. *Consumed: Why Americans Love, Hate, and Fear Food.* New York: Simon & Schuster, 1994.

BODY IMAGE

Dixon, M. *Love the Body You Were Born With.* New York: Perigee, 1996.

Freedman, R. *Bodylove.* New York: Perennial Library, 1988.

Goodman, W. C. *The Invisible Woman.* Carlsbad, Calif.: Gurze Books, 1995.

Hall., L., and Cohn, L. *Self-Esteem: Tools for Recovery.* Carlsbad, Calif.: Gurze Books, 1990.

Hutchinson, M. G. *Transforming Body Image.* Freedom, Calif.: The Crossing Press, 1985.

Johnson, C. A. *Self-Esteem Comes in All Sizes.* New York: Doubleday, 1995.

Johnston, J. E. *Appearance Obsession.* Deerfield Beach, Fla.: Health Communications, 1994.

Rodin, J. *Body Traps.* New York: Quill, 1992.

Schroeder, C. R. *Fat Is Not a Four-Letter Word.* Minneapolis: Chronimed, 1992.

Sied, R. P. *Never Too Thin: Why Women Are At War With Their Bodies.* New York: Prentice-Hall, 1989.

Wolf, N. *The Beauty Myth.* New York: Anchor, 1991.

Zerbe, K. J. *The Body Betrayed.* Carlsbad, Calif.: Gurze Books, 1993.

The Nondieting Approach

Foreyt, J. P., and G. K. Goodrick. *Living Without Dieting*. New York: Warner, 1992.

Fraser, L. *Losing It: America's Obsession with Weight and the Industry That Feeds It*. New York: Dutton, 1997.

Gaesser, G. *Big Fat Lies*. New York: Fawcett Columbine, 1996.

Hall, L. *Full Lives: Women Who Have Freed Themselves from Weight Obsessions*. Carlsbad, Calif.: Gurze Books, 1993.

Hirschmann, J. R., and C. H. Munter. *Overcoming Overeating*. New York: Fawcett Columbine, 1988.

Hirschmann, J. R., and C. H. Munter. *When Women Stop Hating Their Bodies*. New York: Fawcett Columbine, 1995.

Kano, S. *Making Peace with Food*. New York: Perennial Library, 1989.

Latimer, J. L. *Beyond the Food Game*. Denver: Living Quest, 1993.

Roth, G. *When You Eat at the Refrigerator, Pull Up a Chair*. New York: Hyperion, 1998.

Roth, G. *Appetites*. New York: Plume, 1997.

Roth, G. *Breaking Free from Compulsive Eating*. New York: Plume, 1993.

Roth, G. *Feeding the Hungry Heart*. New York: Plume, 1993.

Roth, G. *When Food Is Love*. New York: Plume, 1992.

Tribole, E., and E. Resch. *Intuitive Eating*. New York: St. Martin's Press, 1995.

Waterhouse, D. *Like Mother, Like Daughter*. New York: Hyperion, 1997.

Waterhouse, D. *Outsmarting the Female Fat Cell*. New York: Warner, 1993.

Waterhouse, D. *Why Women Need Chocolate*. New York: Hyperion, 1995.

Mind-Body and Alternative Medicine

Benson, H. *Beyond the Relaxation Response*. New York: Times Books, 1984.

Benson, H. *The Relaxation Response*. New York: Avon, 1975.

Benson, H. *Timeless Healing*. New York: Scribner, 1996.

Berry, C. R. *Is Your Body Trying To Tell You Something?* Berkeley, Calif.: Page Mill Press, 1997.

Borysenko, J. *A Woman's Life*. New York: Riverhead, 1996.

Borysenko, J. *Minding the Body, Mending the Mind*. New York: Bantam Books, 1987.

Carlson, R. *Don't Sweat the Small Stuff . . . And It's All Small Stuff*. New York: Hyperion, 1997.

Carper, J. *Miracle Cures*. New York: HarperCollins, 1997.

Chopra, D. *Ageless Body, Timeless Mind*. New York: Harmony, 1993.

Domar, A. *Healing Mind, Healthy Woman*. New York: Delta, 1996.

Elias, J., and S. R. Masline. *Healing Herbal Remedies*. New York: Dell, 1995.

Kabat-Zinn, J. *Wherever You Go, There You Are*. New York: Hyperion, 1994.

McIntyre, A. *The Complete Woman's Herbal*. New York: Henry Holt, 1994.

Morton, M., and M. Morton. *Five Steps to Selecting the Best Alternative Medicine*. Novato, Calif.: New World Library, 1996.

Tyler, V. *The Honest Herbal*. Binghamton, N.Y.: Hawthorn Press, 1993.

Weil, A. *Eight Weeks to Optimal Healing*. New York: Knopf, 1997.

Weil, A. *Natural Health, Natural Medicine*. New York: Houghton Mifflin, 1995.

Weil, A. *Spontaneous Healing*. New York: Knopf, 1995

NEWSLETTERS

Dr. Christiane Northrup's Health Wisdom for Women
Phillips Publishing
P.O. Box 60110
Potomac, MD 20897
800-804-0935

A Friend Indeed: For Women in the Prime of Life
Box 1710
Champlain, NY 12919
514-843-5730

Harvard Women's Health Watch
164 Longwood Avenue
Boston, MA 02115
617-432-1485

Hot Flash: Newsletter for Midlife and Older Women
P.O. Box 816
Stony Brook, NY 11790

Menopause News
2074 Union Street
San Francisco, CA 94123
800-241-6366

Midlife Wellness
Center for Climacteric Studies
University of Florida
901 N.W. 8th Avenue, Suite B1
Gainesville, FL 32061

Women's Health Connection
P.O. Box 6338
Madison, WI 53716
800-366-6632

Woman's Health Advocate Newsletter
P.O. Box 420235
Palm Coast, FL 32142
800-829-5876

ORGANIZATIONS

American Dietetic Association
216 West Jackson Boulevard
Chicago, IL 60606
800-877-1600 ext. 5800

Center for Climacteric Studies
University of Florida
901 N.W. 8th Avenue, Suite B1
Gainesville, FL 32061

Largely Positive
P.O. Box 17223
Glendale, WI 52317

The Melpomene Institute
1010 University Avenue
St. Paul, MN 55104
612-642-1951

National Association to Advance Fat Acceptance (NAAFA)
P.O. Box 188620
Sacramento, CA 95818
800-442-1214

The National Center for Overcoming Overeating
P. O. Box 1257
Old Chelsea Station
New York, NY 10113
212-875-0442

National Osteoporosis Foundation
1150 17th Street, N.W., Suite 500
Washington, DC 20036
202-223 2226

North American Menopause Society
P.O. Box 94527
Cleveland, OH 44101
216-844-8748

Women's Health America
P.O. Box 259690
Madison, WI 53725
800-558-7046

Women Insisting on Natural Shapes (WINS)
P.O. Box 19938
Sacramento, CA 95819
800-600-9467

Adlercreutz, H., et al. 1991. Urinary excretion of ligans and isoflavenoid phytoestrogens in Japanese men and women consuming a traditional Japanese diet. *Am J Clin Nutr* 54:1093.

Adlercreutz, H., et al. 1992. Dietary phytoestrogens and the menopause in Japan. *Lancet* 339:1233.

Allred, J. B. 1995. Too much of a good thing: an overemphasis on eating low fat may be contributing to the alarming increase in overweight among adults. *J Am Dietet Assoc* 95:417.

Anderson, B., et al. 1990. Influence of menopause on dietary treatment of obesity. *J Intern Med* 227:173.

Anderson, J. W., et al. 1995. Meta-analysis of the effects of soy protein intake on serum lipids. *New Eng J Med* 333:276.

Arciero, P. J., et al. 1993. Resting metabolic rate is lower in women than in men. *J Appl Physiol* 75:2514.

Auld, G. W., et al. 1991. Gender differences in adults' knowledge about fat and cholesterol. *J Am Diet Assoc* 91:1391.

Avis, N. E., et al. 1991. A longitudinal analysis of women's attitudes toward the menopause: results from the Massachusetts Women's Health Study. *Maturitas* 13:65.

Backstrom, T. 1992. Neuroendocrinology of premenstrual syndrome. *Clin Obstet & Gynecol* 35:612.

Barish, E. B. 1994. Dieting may be a losing proposition. *Harvard Health Letter* (August):4.

Barlow, C. E., et al. 1995. Physical fitness, mortality, and obesity. *Int J Obesity* 9:S41.

Baron-Faust, R. 1997. Welcome to perimenopause. *American Health* (January/February):68.

Barr, S. I., et al. 1994. Restrained eating and ovulatory disturbances: possible implications for bone health. *Am J Clin Nutr* 59:92.

Barrett-Connor, E. 1991. Postmenopausal estrogen and prevention bias. *Annals Int Med* 115:455.

Bates, C. D. 1997. Protein propaganda. *Shape Magazine* (April):135.

Baumgartner, R. N., et al. 1996. Associations of fat and muscle masses with bone mineral in elderly men and women. *Am J Clin Nutr* 63:365.

Blair, S. N., et al. 1989. Physical fitness and all-cause mortality: a prospective study of healthy men and women. *JAMA* 262:2395.

Blair, S. N., et al. 1995. Changes in physical fitness and all-cause mortality: a prospective study of healthy and unhealthy men. *JAMA* 273:1093.

Blundell, J. E. 1992. Serotonin and the biology of feeding. *Am J Clin Nutr* 55:155S.

Borysenko, J. 1987. *Minding the Body, Mending the Mind* New York: Bantam Books.

Bouchard, C. 1991. Current understanding of the etiology of obesity: genetic and nongenetic factors. *Am J Clin Nutr* 55:1561S.

Bouchard, C., et al. 1988. Inheritance of the amount and distribution of human body fat. *Int J Obesity* 12:205.

Bowen, S. A. A., et al. 1993. Influences of eating patterns on change to a low-fat diet. *J Am Diet Assoc* 93:1309.

Brandi, M. L. 1992. Flavoids: biochemical effects on therapeutic applications. *Bone and Mineral* 19:S3.

Brody, L. 1997. Dieting on the dark side. *Shape Magazine* (March):108.

Brownwell, K. 1991. Dieting and the search for the perfect body: where physiology and culture collide. *Behavior Therapy* 22:1.

Brownwell, K. D., et al. 1994. Medical, metabolic, and physiological effects of weight cycling. *Arch Intern Med* 154:1325.

Brownwell, K. D., et al. 1994. The dieting maelstrom: is it possible and advisable to lose weight? *Am Psychol* 40:781.

Caffeine: not so bad for your bones after all. 1997. *Tufts University Diet and Nutrition Letter* (September):1.

Caputo, F. A., et al. 1993. Human dietary responses to perceived manipulation of fat content in a midday meal. *Int J Obes Related Metab Discord* 17:237.

Carlson, K. J., et al. 1994. The Maine Women's Health Study: outcomes of hysterectomy. *Obstet & Gynecol* 83:556.

Carrier, K. M. 1994. Rethinking traditional weight management programs: a 3 year follow-up evaluation of a new approach. *J Psychol* 128:517.

Cash, T. F., et al. 1986. The great American shape-up. *Psychol Today* (April):30.

Cassel, J. 1995. Social anthropology and nutrition: a different look at obesity in America. *J Am Diet Assoc* 95:424.

Cauley, J. A., et al. 1989. The epidemiology of serum sex hormones in postmenopausal women. *Am J Epidem* 129:1120.

Chromium picolinate claims thin on evidence. 1995. *Tufts University Diet and Nutrition Letter* 13:2.

Cross, A. T., et al. 1994. Snacking patterns among 1800 adults and children. *J Am Diet Assoc* 94:1398.

Den Tonkelaar, I., et al. 1989. Factors influencing waist/hip ratio in randomly selected pre- and post-menopausal women in the DOM-project. *Int J Obesity* 13:817.

Domar, A. 1996. *Healing Mind, Healthy Woman* New York: Delta.

Drewnowski, A. 1997. Why do we like fat? *J Am Diet Assoc* 97: S58.

Drewnowski, A., et al. 1987. Men and body image: are men satisfied with their body weight? *Psychsomatic Med* 49:626.

Drinkwater, B. 1995. Why women should lift weights. *Women's Health Digest* 1:137.

Drinkwater, B. L., et al. 1984. Bone mineral content of amenorrheic and eumenorrheic athletes. *New Eng J Med* 311:277.

Dugdale, A. E., et al. 1989. The effect of lactation and other factors on post-partum changes in body weight and triceps skinfold thickness. *Br J Nutr* 61:149.

Dumesic, D., et al. 1993. Obesity affects circulating estradiol levels in premenopausal women receiving leuprolide acetate depot. *Int J Fertil* 38:139.

Dunn, L., et al. 1997. Does estrogen prevent aging skin? *Arch Dermatol* 133:339.

Dying to be perfect. 1997. *Women's Health Advocate* (February):5.

Egeland, G. M., et al. 1990. Hormone replacement therapy and lipoprotein changes during early menopause. *Obstet and Gynecol* 76:776.

Evans, M., and A. Shakeshaft. 1996. *The Noisy Passage*. Bridgeport, Conn.: Hysteria Publications.

Evans, W. J., et al. 1997. Nutrition, exercise, and healthy aging. *J Am Diet Assoc* 97:632.

Experts urge testing for sluggish thyroid. 1997. *Tufts University Diet and Nutrition Letter* (March):1.

Exercise for what ails you. 1997. *Harvard Health Letter* (March):8.

Fat chance. 1997. *Nutrition Action Healthletter* (May):2.

Fat free foods: a dieter's downfall. 1995. *Environmental Nutrition* 18:4.

Ferraro, R., et al. 1992. Lower sedentary metabolic rates in women compared with men. *J Clin Invest* 90:780.

Folsom, A. R., et al. 1993. Body fat distribution and 5 year risk of death in older women. *JAMA* 269:483.

Foltin, R. W., et al. 1990. Caloric compensation for lunches varying in fat and carbohydrate content by humans in a residential laboratory. *Am J Clin Nutr* 52:969.

Fontaine, K. L. 1991. The conspiracy of culture: women's issues in body size. *Nursing Clinics of North Am* 26:669.

Foreyt, J. P., et al. 1993. Evidence for success of behavior modification in weight loss and control. *Ann Intern Med* 119:698.

Foreyt, J. P., et al. 1993. Weight management without dieting. *Nutr Today* (March/April):4.

Fornari, V., et al. 1994. Anorexia nervosa: "thirty something." *J Substance Abuse Treatment* 11:45.

Franklin, D. 1996. The healthiest women in the world. *Health* (September):56.

Fraser, L. 1997. *Losing It.* New York: Dutton.

Freedman, R. R., et al. 1992. Behavioral treatment of menopausal hot flashes: evaluation by ambulatory monitoring. *Am J Obstet Gynecol* 167:436.

Fukagawa, N. K., et al. 1990. Effect of age on body composition and resting metabolic rate. *Am J Physiol* 259: E233.

Gaesser, G. A. 1996. *Big Fat Lies.* New York: Fawcett Columbine.

Gallup Organization. 1990. Gallup survey of public opinion regarding diet and health. Prepared for the American Dietetic Association. Princeton, N.J.

Gallup Organization. 1993. Women's knowledge and behavior regarding health and fitness. Conducted for the American Dietetic Association and Weight Watchers (June).

Gardner, A. W., et al. 1993. Physical activity is a significant predictor of body density in women. *Am J Clin Nutr* 57:8.

Garner, D. M., et al. 1991. Confronting the failure of behavioral and dietary treatment for obesity. *Clin Psychol Rev* 11:729.

Geliebter, A., et al. 1996. Reduced stomach capacity in obese subjects after dieting. *Am J Clin Nutr* 63:170.

Glatzer, R. 1997. Living to 100. *American Health* (July):56.

Golay, A., et al. 1996. Similar weight loss with low or high carbohydrate diets. *Am J Clin Nutr* 63:174.

Goldstein, D. J. 1992. Beneficial health effects of modest weight loss. *Int J Obesity Related Metabolic Disorders* 16:397.

Gortmaker, S. L., et al. 1990. Inactivity, diet, and the fattening of America. *J Am Diet Assoc* 90:1247.

Gosden, R. G. 1985. *Biology of Menopause*. London: Academic Press.

Green, M. W., et al. 1995. Impaired cognitive functioning in dieters during dieting. *Psychol Med* 25:1003.

Grilo, C. M. 1995. The role of physical activity in weight loss and weight loss maintenance. *Med Exerc Nutr Health* 4:60.

Guicheney, P., et al. 1988. Platelet serotonin content and plasma tryptophan in peri- and postmenopausal women: variations with plasma oestrogen levels and depressive symptoms. *Euro J Clin Invest* 18:297.

Haarbo, J., et al. 1991. Postmenopausal hormone replacement therapy prevents central distribution of body fat after menopause. *Metabolism* 40:1323.

Haffner, S., et al. 1991. Increased upper body and overall adiposity is associated with decreased sex hormone binding globulin in postmenopausal women. *Int J Obesity* 15:471.

Haines, P. A., et al. 1992. Eating patterns and energy and nutrient intake of U.S. women. *J Am Diet Assoc* 92:698.

Hales, D. 1997. The joy of midlife sex. *American Health* (January):78.

Hallmark, M. A., et al. 1996. Effects of chromium and resistance training on muscle strength and body composition. *Med Sci Sports Exerc* (January):139.

Hammar, M., et al. 1990. Does physical exercise influence the frequency of hot flashes? *Acta Obstet Gynecol Scand* 69:409

Hammond, C. B. 1996. Menopause and hormone replacement therapy: an overview. *Obstet & Gynecol* 87:2S.

Harris, T. B., et al. 1993. Overweight, weight loss, and coronary heart disease in older women. *Am J Epidem* 137:1318.

Howat, P. M., et al. 1989. The influence of diet, body fat, menstrual cycling, and activity upon the bone density of females. *J Am Diet Assoc* 89:1305.

Hunter, D. J., et al. 1996. Cohort studies of fat intake and the risk of breast cancer. *New Eng J Med* 334:356.

Hutchins, A. 1995. Fruits, vegetables, and legumes: effect of urinary isoflavonoid phytoestrogen and ligin excretion. *J Am Diet Assoc* 95:769.

If you are born to hate broccoli. 1997. *Health* (May):11.

Jaret, P. 1997. Choose treatments you believe in. *Health* (April):99.

Jenkins, D. J. A., et al. 1989. Nibbling versus gorging: metabolic advantages of increased meal frequency. *N Engl J Med* 321:929.

Jensen, J., et al. 1986. Estrogen-progesterone replacement therapy changes body composition in early postmenopausal women. *Maturitas* 8:209.

Johnson, B. 1997. *Living Somewhere Between Estrogen and Death*. Dallas, Tex.: Word Publishing.

Kanazawa, T. 1995. Soy and heart disease prevention. *J Nutr* 125:639S.

Kaym S., et al. 1991. Associations of body mass and fat distribution with sex hormone concentrations in postmenopausal women. *Int J Epidemiol* 20:151.

Kawachi, I., et al. 1996. A prospective study of coffee drinking and suicide in women. *Arch Intern Med* 156:521.

Keller, H. H. 1995. Weight gain impacts morbidity and mortality in institutionalized older persons. *J Am Geriatrics Soc* 43:165.

Kennedy, A. 1995. The evidence for soybean products as cancer preventive agents. *J Nutr* 125:733S.

King, G. A., et al. 1987. Food perceptions in dieters and nondieters. *Appetite* 8:147.

Kirschner. M. A., et al. 1990. Androgen-estrogen metabolism in women with upper body vs. lower body obesity. *J Clin Endocrinol Metab* 70:473.

Knight, D. C., et al. 1996. A review of the clinical effects of phytoestrogens. *Obstet & Gynecol* 87:897.

Kohrt, W. M., et al. 1992. Exercise training improves fat distribution patterns in 60- to 70-year-old men and women. *J Gerontol* 47: M99.

Kohrt, W. M., et al. 1992. Body composition of healthy sedentary and trained, young and older women. *Med Sci Sports Exerc* 24:832.

Krall, E. A., et al. 1994. Walking is related to bone density and rates of bone loss. *Am J Med* 96:20.

Kramer, F. M., et al. 1989. Long-term follow-up of behavioral treatment of obesity: patterns of regain among men and women. *Int J Obesity* 13:123.

Kretsch, M. J., et al. 1997. Cognitive effects of a long-term weight reducing diet. *Int J Obesity* 21:14.

Kritz-Silverstein, D., et al. 1996. Long-term postmenopausal hormone use, obesity, and body fat distribution in older women. *JAMA* 275:46.

Kuczmarski, R. J., et al. 1994. Increasing prevalence of overweight among U.S. adults. *JAMA* 272:205.

Langois, J. A., et al. 1996. Weight change between age 50 and old age is associated with risk of hip fracture in white women age 67 and older. *Archives Int Med* 156:989.

Lapidus, L., et al. 1989. Obesity, adipose tissue distribution and health in women—results from a population study in Gothenburg, Sweden. *Appetite* 12:25.

Ley, C. J. at al. 1992. Sex and menopausal associated changes in body fat distribution. *Am J Clin Nutr* 55:950.

Leibel, R. L., et al. 1995. Changes in energy expenditure resulting from altered body weight. *New Eng J Med* 332:621.

Leiblum, S. R., et al. 1986. Women's attitudes toward the menopause: an update. *Maturitis* 8:47.

Liebman, B., et al. 1996. One size does not fit all. *Nutrition Action Healthletter* (November):10.

Lissner, L., et al. 1991. Variability of body weight and health outcomes in the Framingham population. *New Eng J Med* 324:1839.

Lock, M. 1994. Menopause in cultural context. *Exp Gerontol* 29:307.

Lock M., et al. 1989. Cultural construction of the menopausal syndrome: the Japanese case. *Maturitas* 10:317.

Losonczy, K. G., et al. 1995. Does weight loss from middle age to old age explain the inverse weight mortality in old age? *Am J Epidem* 141:312.

Love, S. 1997. *Dr. Susan Love's Hormone Book* New York: Random House.

Manson, J. E., at al. 1995. Body weight and mortality among women. *N Engl J Med* 333:677.

Marano, H. E. 1993. Chemistry and craving. *Psychol Today* (January):30.

Martin, M. C., et al. 1993. Menopause without symptoms: the endocrinology of menopause among rural Mayan Indians. *Am J Obstet Gynecol* 168:1839.

Martini, M. C., et al. 1994. Effect of menstrual cycle on energy and nutrient intake. *Am J Clin Nutr* 60:895.

Matthews, K., et al. 1990. Influences of natural menopause on psychological characteristics and symptoms of middle-aged healthy women. *J Consult Clin Psychol* 58:345.

Matthews, K. A. 1992. Myths and realities of menopause. *Psychosomatic Med* 54:1.

Matthews, K. A., et al. 1989. Menopause and risk factors for coronary heart disease. *New Engl J Med* 321:641.

McCarger, L. J., et al. 1991. The effect of weight cycling on metabolism. *J Can Diet Assoc* 54:138.

McKinlay, J. B., et al. 1989. The questionable physiologic and epidemiologic basis for a male climacteric syndrome: preliminary results from the Massachusetts Male Aging Study. *Maturitas* 11:103.

McNaughton, J. P. 1991. Eating styles of U.S. women. *Food and Nutrition News* 63:11.

McNutt, K. 1997. What's bothering Olestra opponents? *Nutrition Today* 32:41.

Meskin, M. S. 1995. Potential dangers of herbal and herb-related products. *Nutrition and the MD* (February):5.

Messina, M. 1991. The role of soy products in reducing risk of cancer. *J Nat Cancer Instit* 83:541.

Middle age spread. 1995. *Harvard Women's Health Watch* (August):6.

Miller, W. C., et al. 1990. Diet composition, energy intake, and exercise in relation to body fat in men and women. *Am J Clin Nutr* 52:426.

Ming-Xin, T., et al. 1996. Effect of oestrogen during menopause on risk and age at onset of Alzheimer's disease. *Lancet* 348:429.

Morris, A., et al. 1989. The changing shape of female models. *Int J Eating Disorders* 8:593.

Murkies, A. L. 1995. Dietary flour supplementation decreases postmenopausal hot flashes: effect of soy and wheat. *Maturitas* 21:189.

Nelson, M. 1997. *Strong Women Stay Young.* New York: Bantam Books.

Nelson, M. E., et al. 1994. Effects of high-intensity strength training on multiple risk factors for osteoporotic fractures. *JAMA* 272:1909.

Neumark-Sztainer, D., et al. 1995. Dieting and binge eating: which dieters are at risk? *J Am Diet Assoc* 95:586.

Newsbreaks: men overeat for different reasons than women. 1997. *Nutrition Today* 32:4.

Oliwenstein, L. 1997. The great debate: protein vs. carbohydrates. *Living Fit* (March):75.

Parham, E. S. 1996. Is there a new weight paradigm? *Nutrition Today* 31:155.

Pasquali, R., et al. 1994. Body weight, fat distribution and the menopausal status in women. *Int J Obesity* 18:614.

Poehlman, E. T., et al. 1993. Metabolic determinants of the decline of resting metabolic rate in aging females. *Am J Physiol* 75:2514.

Poehlman, E. T., et al. 1995. Physiological predictors of increasing total and central adiposity in aging men and women. *Archives Int Med* 155:2443.

Poehlman, E. T., et al. 1995. Changes in energy balance and body composition at menopause: a controlled longitudinal study. *Annals of Int Med* 123:673.

Polivy, J. 1996. Psychological consequences of food restriction. *J Am Dietet Assoc* 96:589.

Polivy, J., et al. 1992. Undieting: a program to help people stop dieting. *Int J Eating Disorders* 11:261.

Posner, B. M., et al. 1995. Secular trends in diet and risk factors of cardiovascular disease: The Framingham Study. *J Am Diet Assoc* 95:171.

Powell, J. J., et al. 1994. The effects of different percentages of dietary fat intake, exercise, and caloric restriction on body composition and body weight in obese women. *Am J Health Promotion* 8:442.

Prince, R. L., et al. 1991. Prevention of postmenopausal osteoporosis. *New Eng J Med* 325:1189.

Raison, J., et al. 1988. Regional differences in adipose tissue lipoprotein lipase in relation to body fat distribution and menopausal status in obese women. *Int J Obesity* 12:465.

Rebuffe-Scrive, M., et al. 1985. Fat cell metabolism in different regions in women. *Am J Clin Nutr* 28:445.

Rebuffe-Scrive, M., et al. 1986. Metabolism of mammary, abdominal, and femoral adipocytes in women before and after menopause. *Metabolism* 35:792.

Rebuffe-Scrive, M., et al. 1987. Regional adipose tissue metabolism in men and postmenopausal women. *Int J Obesity* 11:347.

Rodin, J., et al. 1990. Weight cycling and fat distribution. *Int J Obesity* 14:303.

Rodin, J., et al. 1991. Food cravings in relationship to body mass index, restraint, and estradiol levels. *Appetite* 17:177.

Rolls, B. J., et al. 1991. Gender differences in eating behavior and body weight regulation. *Health Psychol* 10:133.

Rolls, B. J., et al. 1994. Satiety after preloads with different amounts of fat and carbohydrate: implications for obesity. *Am J Clin Nutr* 60:476.

Roughan, P., et al. 1990. Long-term effects of a physiologically based group programme for women preoccupied with weight and eating behavior. *Int J Obesity* 14:135.

Roust, L. R., et al. 1994. Effects of isoenergetic, low-fat diets on energy metabolism in lean and obese women. *Am J Clin Nutr* 60:470.

Saab, P. G., et al. 1989. Premenopausal and postmenopausal women differ in their cardiovascular and neuroendocrine responses to stress. *Psychophysiology* 26:270.

Schwartz, M. W., et al. 1997. The new biology of body weight regulation. *J Am Diet Assoc* 97:54.

Second Time Around: weight study gets pounded. 1995. *Women's Health Advocate Newsletter* 2:6.

Seidell, J. C., et al. 1996. Overweight, underweight, and mortality: a prospective study of 48,287 men and women. *Archives Int Med* 156:958.

Serdula, M. K., et al. 1995. Fruit and vegetable intake among adults in 16 states: results of a brief telephone survey. *Am J Pub Health* 85:236

Shapiro, L., et al. 1997. Is fat that bad? *Newsweek* (April):58.

Sherwin, B. B. 1994. Estrogenic effects in memory in women. *Ann NY Acad Sci* 14:213.

Shide, D. J., et al. 1995. Information about the fat content of preloads influences energy intake in healthy women. *J Am Diet Assoc* 95:993.

Shimokata, H., et al. 1989. Studies in the distribution of body fat: effects of age, sex, and obesity. *J Gerontol* 44: M66.

Silver, A. J., et al. 1993. Effect of aging on body fat. *J Am Geriatr Soc* 41:211.

Simpson, E. 1989. Regulation of estrogen biosynthesis by human adipose cells. *Endocrin Rev* 10:136.

Skender, M. L., et al. 1996. Comparison of 2-year weight loss trends in behavioral treatments of obesity: diet, exercise, and combined interventions. *J Am Diet Assoc* 96:342.

Smith, D. E., et al. 1994. Longitudinal changes in adiposity associated with pregnancy. *JAMA* 271:1747.

Smith, W. P., et al. 1995. Meditation as an adjunct to a happiness enhancement program. *J Clin Psychol* 51:269.

Somer, E. 1996. Diets are for dummies. *Shape* (November):87.

St. Jeor, S. T. 1993. The role of weight management in the health of women. *J Am Diet Assoc* 93:1007.

Stampler, M. J., et al. 1991. Postmenopausal estrogen therapy and cardiovascular risk. *New Eng J Med* 325:756.

Stratakis, C. A., et al. 1995. Neuroendocrinology and the pathophysiology of the stress system. *Ann N. Y. Acad Sci* (December):1.

Striegel-Moore, R., et al. 1986. Psychological and behavioral correlates of feeling fat in women. *Int J Eating Disorders* 5:935.

Telsh, C. F., et al. 1993. The effects of a very low calorie diet on binge eating. *Behav Therapy* 24:177.

The wellness guide to herbal medicines. 1997. *UC Berkeley Wellness Letter* (September):4.

Thompson, J. K. 1986. Larger than life. *Psychol Today* (April):38.

Thorton, B., et al. 1991. Gender role tying, the superwoman ideal and the potential for eating disorders. *Sex Roles* 25:469.

Too much exercise coupled with too few calories challenges immune function. 1995. *Environmental Nutr* (January):8.

Troiano, R. P., et al. 1996. The relationship between body weight and mortality: a quantitative analysis of combined information from existing studies. *Int J Obesity* 20:63.

Tyler, V. 1993. *The Honest Herbal* Binghamton, N.Y.: Hawthorn Press.

Ushiroyama, T., et al. 1995. Endocrine function of the peri- and postmenopausal ovary. *Hormone Research* 44:64.

Van Gaal, L., et al. 1995. Lipid and lipoprotein changes after long-term weight reduction: the influence of gender and body fat distribution. *J Am College Nutr* 14:382.

Wang, C. 1994. Ligans and flavonoids inhibit aromatase enzyme in human preadipocytes. *J Steroid Biochem Mol Biol* 50:205.

Wang, Q., et al. 1994. Total and regional body composition changes in early postmenopausal women: age-related or menopause-related? *Am J Clin Nutr* 160:843.

Wardle, J., et al. 1988. Control and loss of control over eating: an experimental investigation. *J Abnormal Psychol* 94:78.

Watson, T., et al. 1996. Are you too fat? *US News and World Report* (January) 8:52.

Webb, D. 1995. Does pasta make you fat? *American Health* (October):80.

Webb, P. 1986. 24 hour energy expenditure and the menstrual cycle. *Am J Clin Nutr* 44:614.

Weight loss news that's easy to swallow. 1996. *Tufts University Diet and Nutrition Letter* (April):1.

What is a reasonable weight loss? 1997. *Eating Disorders Review* (March):5.

White, J. H. 1991. Feminism, eating, and mental health. *Adv Nurs Sci* 13:68.

Wilcox, G., et al. 1990. Oestrogenic effects of plant foods in post-menopausal women. *Brit Med J* 301:905.

Willett, W. C., et al. 1995. Weight, weight change, and coronary heart disease in women. *JAMA* 273:461.

Williamson, D. F., et al. 1990. The 10 year incidence of overweight and major weight gain in U.S. adults. *Arch Intern Med* 150:665.

Williamson, D. F., et al. 1991. The 10 year incidence of obesity and major weight gain in black and white U.S. women age 30 to 55 years. *Am J Clin Nutr* 53:1515S.

Williamson, D. F., et al. 1992. Weight loss attempts in adults: Goals, duration, and rate of weight loss. *Am J Public Health* 82:1251.

Wing, R. R., et al. 1991. Weight gain at the time of menopause. *Arch. Intern. Med* 151:97.

Wing, R. R., et al. 1992. Change in waist-hip ratio with weight loss and its association with change in cardiovascular risk factors. *Am J Clin Nutr* 55:1086.

Wing, R. R., et al. 1995. Effect of modest weight loss on changes in cardiovascular risk factors: are there differences between men and women or between weight loss and maintenance? *Int J Obesity.* 19:67.

Wood, M. 1995. Weight loss: a sex-linked trait. *Agricultural Research* (August):14.

Wooley, S. C., et al. 1984. Feeling fat in a thin society. *Glamour* (February):198.

Wren, B. G., and L. E. Nachtigall. 1996. *Clinical Management of the Menopause*. Sidney, Austalia: McGraw-Hill.

Wyon, Y., et al. 1995. Effects of acupuncture on climacteric vasomotor symptoms, quality of life, and urinary excretion of neuropeptides among postmenopausal women. *Menopause* 2:3.

Zamboni, M., et al. 1992. Body fat distribution in pre- and post-menopausal women: metabolic and anthropometric variables in the interrelationships. *Int J Obesity* 16:495.

Index

Debra Waterhouse, M.P.H., R.D., is an internationally recognized nutritionist and best-selling author of *Outsmarting the Female Fat Cell*, *Why Women Need Chocolate*, and *Like Mother, Like Daughter*. She received her undergraduate degree from Simmons College in Boston and her advanced degree from the University of California at Berkeley. As an expert in women's health and a leader in the antidieting movement, she has been featured on numerous radio and television programs, including *Dateline*, *Good Morning America*, and *CBS This Morning*, and on CNN. Through her private practice, seminars, and workshops, she has inspired hundreds of thousands of women to accept the realities of their female bodies and embrace a natural, nonrestrictive approach to eating and weight control. It's a formula that has worked for her. Once a food-preoccupied, yo-yo dieter, she now maintains a comfortable, healthy weight by exercising, trusting her body's messages, and eating her favorite foods—pizza, potato chips, and chocolate—in moderation. Her goal is to help women of all ages break free from body dissatisfaction and food guilt and start feeding and respecting the bodies they were born with. She lives and works in the San Francisco Bay area.